THE TRUTH ABOUT
SUICIDE

THE TRUTH ABOUT SUICIDE

Robert N. Golden, M.D.
University of Wisconsin–Madison
General Editor

Fred L. Peterson, Ph.D.
University of Texas–Austin
General Editor

Donna Holland Barnes, Ph.D.
Principal Author

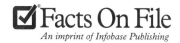

☑ Facts On File
An imprint of Infobase Publishing

The Truth About Suicide

Facts On File, Inc.
An imprint of Infobase Publishing
132 West 31st Street
New York, NY 10001

Library of Congress Cataloging-in-Publication Data

Barnes, Donna Holland.
  The truth about suicide / Robert N. Golden, general editor, Fred L. Peterson, general editor; Donna Holland Barnes, principal author.
     p. cm. − (The truth about)
  Includes index.
  ISBN-13: 978-0-8160-7637-6 (hardcover : alk. paper)
  ISBN-10: 0-8160-7637-5 (hardcover : alk. paper) 1. Suicide. 2. Suicide−Prevention. 3. Suicide−United States. 4. Suicide−United States−Prevention. I. Golden, Robert N. II. Peterson, Fred (Fred L.) III. Title.
  HV6545.B253 2009
  362.28−dc22
                                          2009016624

Facts On File books are available at special discounts when purchased in bulk quantities for businesses, associations, institutions or sales promotions. Please call our Special Sales Department in New York at (212) 967-8800 or (800) 322-8755.

You can find Facts On File on the World Wide Web at http://www.factsonfile.com

Text design by Kerry Casey
Composition by Mary Susan Ryan-Flynn
Cover printed by Art Print, Taylor, PA
Book printed and bound by Maple Press, York, PA
Date printed: January 2010
Printed in the United States of America

10 9 8 7 6 5 4 3 2 1

This book is printed on acid-free paper and contains 30 percent postconsumer recycled content.

CONTENTS

LIST OF ILLUSTRATIONS

PREFACE

The Truth About series—updated and expanded to include 20 volumes—seeks to identify the most pressing health issues and social challenges confronting our nation's youth. Adolescence is the period between the onset of puberty and the attainment of adult roles and responsibilities. Adolescence is also a time of storm, stress, and risk-taking for many young people. During adolescence, a person's health is influenced by biological, psychological, and social factors, all of which interact with one's environment—family, peers, school, and community. It is a time when teenagers experience profound changes.

With the latest available statistics and new insights that have emerged from ongoing research, The Truth About series seeks to help young people build a foundation of information as they face some of the challenges that will affect their health and well-being. These challenges include high-risk behaviors such as alcohol, tobacco, and other drug use; sexual behaviors that can lead to adolescent pregnancy and sexually transmitted diseases (STDs) such as HIV/AIDS; mental health concerns such as depression and suicide; learning disorders and disabilities, which are often associated with school failures and school dropouts; serious family problems, including domestic violence and abuse; and lifestyle factors, which increase adolescents' risk for non-communicable diseases such as diabetes and cardiovascular disease, among others.

Broader underlying factors also influence adolescent health. These include socioeconomic circumstances such as poverty, available health care, and the political and social situations in which young people live. Although these factors can negatively affect adolescent health and well-being as well as school performance, many of these negative health outcomes are preventable with the proper knowledge and information.

With prevention in mind, the writers and editors of each topical volume in The Truth About series have tried to provide cutting-edge information that is supported by research and scientific evidence. Vital facts are presented that inform youth about the challenges experienced during adolescence, while special features seek to dispel common myths and misconceptions. Some of the main topics explored include abuse, alcohol, death and dying, divorce, drugs, eating disorders, family life, fear and depression, rape, sexual behavior and unplanned pregnancy, smoking, and violence. All volumes discuss risk-taking behaviors and their consequences, healthy choices, prevention, available treatments, and where to get help.

In this new edition of the series, we also have added eight new titles in areas of increasing significance to today's youth. ADHD, or attention-deficit/hyperactivity disorder, and learning disorders are diagnosed with increasing frequency, and many students have observed or know of classmates receiving treatment for these conditions, even if they have not themselves received this diagnosis. Gambling is gaining currency in our culture, as casinos open and expand in many parts of the country, and the Internet offers easy access for this addictive behavior. Another consequence of our increasingly "online" society, unfortunately, is the presence of online predators. Environmental hazards represent yet another danger, and it is important to provide unbiased information about this topic to our youth. Suicide, which for many years has been a "silent epidemic," is now gaining recognition as a major public health problem throughout the life span, including the teenage and young adult years. We now also offer an overview of illness and disease in a volume that includes the major conditions of particular interest and concern to youth. In addition to illness, however, it is essential to emphasize health and its promotion, and this is especially apparent in the volumes on physical fitness and stress management.

It is our intent that each book serve as an accessible, authoritative resource to which young people can turn for accurate and meaningful answers to their specific questions. The series can help them research particular problems and provide an up-to-date evidence base. It is also designed with parents, teachers, and counselors in mind so that they have a reliable resource that they can share with youth who seek their guidance.

Finally, we have tried to provide unbiased facts rather than subjective opinions. Our goal is to help elevate the health of the public with an emphasis on its most precious component—our youth. As young people face the challenges of an increasingly complex world, we as educators want them to be armed with the most powerful weapon available—knowledge.

Robert N. Golden, M.D.
Fred L. Peterson, Ph.D.
General Editors

HOW TO USE THIS BOOK

NOTE TO STUDENTS

Knowledge is power. By possessing knowledge you have the ability to make decisions, ask follow-up questions, or know where to go to obtain more information. In the world of health that is power! That is the purpose of this book—to provide you the power you need to obtain unbiased, accurate information and *The Truth About Suicide*.

Topics in each volume of The Truth About are arranged in alphabetical order, from A to Z. Each of these entries defines its topic and explains in detail the particular issue. At the end of most entries are cross-references to related topics. A list of all topics by letter can be found in the table of contents or at the back of the book in the index.

How have these books been compiled? First, the publisher worked with us to identify some of the country's leading authorities on key issues in health education. These individuals were asked to identify some of the major concerns that young people have about such topics. The writers read the literature, spoke with health experts, and incorporated their own life and professional experiences to pull together the most up-to-date information on health issues, particularly those of interest to adolescents and of concern in *Healthy People 2010*.

Throughout the alphabetical entries, the reader will find sidebars that separate fact from fiction. There are question-and-answer boxes that attempt to address the most common questions that youth ask about sensitive topics. In addition, readers will find a special feature called "Teens Speak"—case studies of teens with personal stories related to the topic in hand.

This may be one of the most important books you will ever read. Please share it with your friends, families, teachers, and classmates. Remember, you possess the power to control your future. One way to affect your course is through the acquisition of knowledge. Good luck and keep healthy.

NOTE TO LIBRARIANS

This book, along with the rest of The Truth About series, serves as a wonderful resource for your researchers. It contains a variety of facts, case studies, and further readings that the reader can use to help answer questions, formulate new questions, or determine where to go to find more information. Even though the topics may be considered delicate by some, don't be afraid to ask patrons if they have questions. Feel free to direct them to the appropriate sources, but do not press them if you encounter reluctance. The best we can do as educators is to let young people know that we are there when they need us.

Robert Golden, M.D.
Fred L. Peterson, Ph.D.
General Editors

SUICIDE: NO LONGER A SECRET

When an anxious mother found out that her 15-year-old son was having suicidal thoughts, she took him to a clinic for help. She felt that her son was in need of overnight care. When they told her there were no beds available and to come back in a couple of days, she complied. When she got home, she asked her son if he was going to be all right, and he said that he would be fine. She watched him most of the night and decided to go to sleep. At 4:00 A.M., she heard a thump coming from the attic. She rolled over and went back to sleep. In the morning, when she called for her son to get ready for school, she could not find him. She went up to the attic and found him on the floor with a rope around his neck. He had hanged himself.

Weeks later, when the mother decided to investigate further into her son's surroundings, she found out that he was being bullied at school. Being bullied can be a pathway to suicide because young adults will sometimes become clinically depressed as a result of this behavior. In fact, it is widely held among the experts who study suicide that clinical depression and suicide can be one foreseeable consequence of being bullied.

Every 17 minutes, another life is lost to suicide. Every day, 86 Americans take their own lives, and thousands attempt suicide. Suicide leaves in its wake family and friends who are traumatized, and some have nowhere to turn.

HISTORY

Prior to the 1600s, "committing suicide" was simply recognized as another form of death. According to Dr. Ed Schneidman, founder of the American Association of Suicidology, an individual could harm himself or herself, or commit self-directed violence, but the basic concept of suicide did not exist. Researchers uncovered one of the first recorded incidents of what would be considered a suicide by today's standards in the form of a poem written by an anonymous Egyptian more than 4,000 years ago. The poem was about a dispute the man was having between himself and his soul. He looks out into society and sees nothing but corruption, dishonesty, injustice, and unfaithfulness, and he began having thoughts of suicide—of ending his life. He writes how his soul urges him to enjoy life and not succumb to this deviant way of thinking. It is not clear in the poem whether the man takes his own life or not, but it is clear from this example that the concept of suicidal thoughts have been around for thousands of years.

In ancient times, suicide was viewed differently from culture to culture. In feudal Japan, for example, suicide was viewed as the granting of a principal honor, ridding a family of shame if a member was caught engaging in deviant behavior or committing an illegal act. These cases were thought of as honorable or "honorable suicides." In the Roman Empire, suicide was seen as a glorious demonstration of wisdom. According to many studies, suicide also was honored in pre-Christian Scandinavia. In those times, ending one's life before getting old and feeble was considered dying with dignity. Early 20th-century records tell of Inuit tribes whose elders sacrificed their lives by wandering alone into the freezing countryside when they felt they could no longer be of use to their families. Here, suicide was considered acceptable to avoid the pain of sickness and old age.

Followers of St. Augustine, who was considered an important figure in the development of Western Christianity and was the first to denounce suicide as an unforgivable sin, also viewed suicide as a sin. They considered it a form of murder, thus a violation of one of the Bible's Ten Commandments, *Thou shall not kill.* Many religious leaders promoted this belief in an effort to discourage people from killing themselves as a means of hurrying achievement of eternal bliss. Christian societies, following Augustine, punished suicide victims by denying them a church burial; in some societies, victims' bodies were dragged through the town to humiliate the individual and his or her family. Often, the family was denied all rights to any property the deceased had left behind.

Suicide was not only a sin against church but also became a crime against the state. When men killed themselves, their families were often left behind as a burden to the state, an expense to the taxpayers. According to researchers, as late as 1955, a man was sentenced to two years in prison for attempting suicide in Great Britain. During the 1800s, most penalties for suicides and attempted suicides were waived if the individual was classified as mentally ill. This enabled families to avoid being disgraced. When someone who was considered of sound mind took his or her own life, family members would keep it a secret for fear it would be believed the suicide victim was mentally ill. During those times, mental illness had a great stigma attached to it, and family dignity and reputation held a high priority. Because of this stigma, suicide became taboo in many communities and cultures.

Today, suicide can be discussed openly. Families are no longer publicly disgraced if they suffer a suicide in the family and no longer feel compelled to keep it a secret. Individuals who complete suicide are now seen as victims, not sinners. In fact, it is for this reason that those in the field of suicide prevention and intervention no longer use the term *commit* when speaking of someone who died by suicide. Terms such as *completed suicide, suicided,* or *died by suicide* are preferred, as these are not associated with wrongdoing, such as *committed murder.* Only recently has the knowledge and tools become available to approach suicide as a preventable problem with realistic opportunities to save lives.

SUICIDE PREVENTION MOVEMENT

In 1996, a suicide prevention movement was started when Jerry and Elise Weyrauch were not only devastated but also frustrated over the suicide of their daughter. As they did not see much being done in the realm of suicide prevention, they founded SPAN (Suicide Prevention Advocacy Group). They wanted to bring suicide prevention to the forefront of society's concerns with the hope of preventing some of the more than 30,000 suicides that occur each year.

They took several trips to Washington, D.C., and met with various political officials. As a result of the Weyrauches' efforts, two years after they founded SPAN, Surgeon General Dr. David Satcher produced a Call to Action that would develop a national strategy to prevent suicide. By 2001, a document was drafted that presented 11 goals and 68 objectives. It required that a variety of organizations and individuals commit time and effort to suicide prevention. This represented the first attempt in the United States to prevent suicide through a coordinated approach.

In 1998, after losing his wife to suicide, Reese Butler founded the Kristian Brooks Hope Center (named after his wife) and launched the first national crisis hotline, 1-800-SUICIDE. In 1994, Dale and Darlene Emme's 16-year-old son Mikey died by suicide in Denver, Colorado. The Emmes were going through the healing process when they realized that Mikey's friends were also suffering. His schoolmates would come by the house to visit the Emmes, and a few of them made yellow ribbons, Mikey's favorite color. It was not long after that that Dale and Darlene founded the Yellow Ribbon Suicide Prevention Program. They developed cards with a list of symptoms of suicidal behavior and passed them out at Mikey's school. Today, they have Yellow Ribbon chapters all over the country, which educate schools on how to prevent suicide among children and young adults.

After losing his son Jason to suicide in 1997, Clark Flatt founded the Jason Foundation. He writes in an open letter to the public:

Dear Friend,

Jason was my youngest son. He was an average 16-year-old. He got mostly B's on his report card, and he loved sports. Especially football. He was active in his youth group and he had a lot of friends. Jason was the one who was always up for going places and trying new things. From all appearances . . . my son loved life.

But on July 16th, 1997, everything changed. My son, Jason became a statistic of the silent epidemic of youth suicide. In trying to come to terms with what happened, I began researching youth suicide. The statistics are alarming. Did you know on average, over 100 young people this week will become victims of youth suicide? But—youth suicide can be prevented. . . .

There are several other organizations founded by families who have lost someone to suicide, motivated by the lack of action to help stop such tragedies. Alison Malmon was a freshman at the University of Pennsylvania when she lost her older brother to suicide in 2000. In 2001, she founded Active Minds on Campus; now there are college chapters all over the country to help educate students on suicide and mental disorders. Also in the year 2000, Phil and Donna Satow lost their son Jed to suicide and founded the Jed Foundation, whose programming and resources have helped colleges, students, and parents recognize and address the signs of emotional distress and suicide. Their organization also developed a screening test for depression in college students, which is widely used.

The common thread among each family discussed is that they were all left without a clue as to why their loved ones had committed such an act, and then wanted to prevent others from going through the same thing. Around 1999, the Weyrauches and the Emmes decided to collaborate to combat suicide as an epidemic. Together they formed the National Suicide Prevention Council, an organization that promotes collaboration, working together to save lives.

WARNING SIGNS AND SAVING LIVES

Everyone needs to help prevent suicide because it is society's problem, not just the problem of the victims and their families. If young adults take the initiative to team up and educate themselves both about some of the warning signs of suicidal behavior and about suicide prevention, lives will be saved. At the end of this book, in "Hotlines and Help Sites," readers will find a list of organizations in which teens and parents can get involved and take action. Also, look especially at entries such as "American Foundation of Suicide Prevention," "Biology of Suicidal Behavior," "Risk and Protective Factors for Suicide," "Stress and Suicide," "Suicide Prevention," "Therapies and Psychodynamics," and "Warning Signs."

RISKY BUSINESS SELF-TEST

There are several self-tests for suicide ideations or thoughts. The following questionnaire consists of 10 statements designed to test the intensity of suicidal thoughts. This scale was developed and tested for validity by Dr. M. David Rudd, a professor of psychology at Baylor University in Texas.

Read the questionnaire carefully, and then on a separate sheet of paper, circle the number for each item that best describes the way you have felt over the past week, including today. Circle only one number.

1. I have been thinking of ways to kill myself. (1) Never (2) Infrequently (3) Sometimes (4) Frequently (5) Always

2. I have told someone I want to kill myself. (1) Never (2) Infrequently (3) Sometimes (4) Frequently (5) Always

3. I believe my life will end in suicide. (1) Never (2) Infrequently (3) Sometimes (4) Frequently (5) Always

4. I have made attempts to kill myself. (1) Never (2) Infrequently (3) Sometimes (4) Frequently (5) Always

5. I feel life just isn't worth living. (1) Never (2) Infrequently (3) Sometimes (4) Frequently (5) Always

6. Life is so bad I feel like giving up. (1) Never (2) Infrequently (3) Sometimes (4) Frequently (5) Always

7. I just wish my life would end. (1) Never (2) Infrequently (3) Sometimes (4) Frequently (5) Always

8. It would be better for everyone involved if I were to die. (1) Never (2) Infrequently (3) Sometimes (4) Frequently (5) Always

9. I feel there is no solution to my problems other than taking my own life. (1) Never (2) Infrequently (3) Sometimes (4) Frequently (5) Always

10. I have come close to taking my own life. (1) Never (2) Infrequently (3) Sometimes (4) Frequently (5) Always

Add the numbers you have circled. The lowest number that you can achieve in this scale is 10, and the highest is 50. 10–13 = low risk of suicide; 14–24 = medium risk; and 25–50 = high risk. If you are at medium risk, talk to an adult as soon as possible. If you are at high risk, inform those who are responsible for you, and tell them to set up emergency care immediately. Thoughts of suicide can be treated, and treatment and help are readily available.

A-TO-Z ENTRIES

■ AFRICAN AMERICANS

See: Ethnicity and Suicide

■ ALCOHOL, DRUGS, AND SUICIDE

Having a physical and psychological **addiction** to alcohol and/or **drugs** and the relationship of that dependence to suicide, the act of taking one's own life after long periods of hopelessness. The consumption of these substances is often a contributing factor to suicide.

Alcohol and drug abuse is highly associated with suicide in three ways. First, alcohol and drugs can cause loss of control and are related to suicide attempts and completed suicides. Second, drugs are frequently used for completing suicide or suicide attempts, and the use of drugs is the third most common method to suicide, after firearms and hanging. Third, studies show that alcohol and drug use are associated with suicide because substance abusers appear to have higher incidence of both completed and attempted suicide than nonabusers.

In 2004, Monica Swhan, an associate professor at the Institute of Public Health, collected data from the Youth Violence Survey that was administered to all public school students enrolled in grades 7, 9, and 11/12. She found that 35 percent of 856 adolescent middle-school-aged youth under the age of 13 consumed alcohol and engaged in risky behavior such as suicide attempts. The use of alcohol and drugs increases **depression** or a depressive state of mind. They slow down the thinking process to the point that a teenager will not want to participate in school or extra activities. If that happens, they may begin to fail in school, get in trouble for missing classes—and these events can then make them feel even more depressed.

Q & A

Question: Don't suicides happen fast, and aren't they usually caused by one sudden traumatic event, so that it's hard to stop them?

Answer: Suicides are not sudden, and they rarely occur without some warning. They are seldom the result of a single experience or loss. Often, there are many contributing events and feelings that take place over a period of time. A sudden traumatic event may be the trigger event to cause a person to decide to die by suicide, but it is unlikely the only cause. **Stressors** may have built over time, becoming difficult to bear.

Alcohol-involved youth who show signs of impulsiveness or irritability are at a higher risk of suicide than other youth, according to a study done in 2004 by K. R. Conner and published in the journal *Suicide and Life Threatening Behavior.* Alcohol and other drug abuse are often related to emotional trauma, psychological stress, and other mental health problems. Some teenagers use alcohol and drugs to relieve their emotional pain. This is especially common among runaway and homeless youth, who may be living on the street. The ironic part about using drugs and alcohol to feel better is that it is more likely to increase emotional problems than to provide an escape from them. A person who has thought about suicide may never actually attempt it while sober but may do so while intoxicated. Simply said, alcohol and drugs increase impulsive acts.

Fact Or Fiction?

Beer or wine is safer to drink than liquor.

The Facts: One 12-ounce beer has about the same amount of alcohol as one five-ounce glass of wine or a 1.5-ounce shot of liquor. It is the amount of ethanol consumed that affects a person most, not the type of alcoholic drink. Studies have shown that alcohol use by youth and young adults increases the risk of both fatal and nonfatal injuries. Also, youth who use alcohol before age 15 are four times more likely to become alcohol dependent than adults who begin drinking at age 21. Other consequences of alcohol use by young people include increased risky sexual behaviors, poor school performance, and increased risk of suicide and homicide.

Increased prevention efforts to delay and reduce early alcohol and drug use among youths are needed and may reduce both violence and suicide attempts. Statistics show that abusing alcohol at an early age can cause long-term damage to a person's organs.

Alcohol abuse is a pattern of drinking that results in harm to one's health, relationships, or ability to keep up with schoolwork. Signs of alcohol abuse include failure to fulfill responsibilities at school or home; drinking in dangerous situations such as while driving; having problems with the law; and continued drinking despite problems that are caused or worsened by drinking. Alcohol abuse can lead to alcohol dependence or addiction.

Q & A

Question: How does alcohol affect a person?

Answer: Alcohol affects every organ in the body—the heart, lungs, intestines, liver, kidneys, stomach, and brain. Alcohol is a depressant, or drug that depresses the nervous system. It is rapidly absorbed from the stomach and small intestine into the bloodstream. It is metabolized in the liver by enzymes, which are chemicals that stimulate the breakdown of substances in the body. However, the liver can only metabolize a small amount of alcohol at a time, leaving the excess alcohol to circulate throughout the body. The intensity of the effect of alcohol on the body is directly related to the amount consumed.

Substance abuse among young people is also one of the most significant risk factors for suicidal behavior. When suicide among adolescents increased through the 1960s and 1980s, it was attributed to the rise of alcohol use and the availability of illicit drugs. For instance, in San Diego, California, the occurrence of drug use was reported to be increased and so were teen suicides in that same period. Multiple substance use–of drugs and alcohol–was common among younger suicide victims in San Diego. What happens in such an environment is that frequent drug use and intoxication with alcohol can cause hopelessness and unhappiness, particularly among youth who are lonely and isolated and who express antisocial behavior.

FAMILY DYSFUNCTION

Family dysfunction, as well as a teenager's personality traits, can lead to substance abuse, especially if there is substance abuse among family members. Teenagers are at greater risk or are more vulnerable to drug use if it is used in the family–parents, siblings, cousins. Family is part of every teenager's experience and encompasses nearly the whole range of emotional experience. The relationships between parents and children, sisters and brothers, aunts and uncles should be warm and safe. However, much tension in the family can sometimes arise—driving teenagers to despair and causing a deep sense of anxiety or depression. Some of the most devastating family incidents that can be pathways to suicide attempts or completions are family violence, child abuse, family breakups, and drug and alcohol abuse.

TEENS SPEAK

Drinking Every Day Led to Thoughts of Suicide

At the age of 13, suicide seemed like a good idea to me. I was growing up in an environment where drugs and alcohol were everywhere. We had bottles of booze at home, but not much food. And there were dealers all over the neighborhood. Sometimes I would not see my mom for a week. Being the oldest, I had to take care of my brothers and sisters, which meant getting them ready for school every day. It made me angry, because I knew my mother was a drug addict. It was her job to take care of us, and she wasn't! Alcohol seemed like a good solution. I just wanted to relax. But when I would get drunk, there were several times when I put a gun in my mouth, wishing I were dead. The constant drinking caused more pain inside.

Luckily, my grandmother came to the rescue. She took me and my younger sisters and brothers to her house to live with her. She let us be kids and took us to church. We discovered spirituality and community. She also helped me get therapy. Psychological counseling and my grandmother's support changed my life and gave me the hope and values that I needed to stay alive.

Generally, these are the behaviors that are associated with severe or acute alcohol use, and that in turn can lead to suicidal behavior:

1. depression and hopelessness
2. aggression

3. narrow-mindedness and narrowing attention to your state of mind

4. poor coping skills or problem-solving techniques.

See also: Culture and Suicide; Families and Other Survivors

FURTHER READING

Bonnie R. J., and M. E. O'Connell, eds. *Reducing Underage Drinking: A Collective Responsibility.* Washington, D.C.: National Academies Press, 2004.

Monti, Peter M., Suzanne M. Colby, and Tracy A. O'Leary, eds. *Adolescents, Alcohol, and Substance Abuse: Reaching Teens through Brief Interventions.* New York: The Guilford Press, 2004.

■ AMERICAN FOUNDATION FOR SUICIDE PREVENTION

A nonprofit organization formed in 1987 by a number of leading experts on suicide, business and community leaders, and survivors of suicide. The founding members believed that only a combined effort would make it possible to fund the research necessary for progress in the prevention of suicide. Such an approach has proven successful with heart disease, cancer, and diabetes, and it was hoped that it would be successful in dealing with **depression** and suicide.

Many of the original founders were concerned with the alarming rise in youth suicide over the past four decades. In the mid-1980s, the suicide of young men had tripled; that of young women had doubled. Suicide is now the second major cause of death among high school and college students. Many of these individuals were **chronically suicidal,** having attempted suicide many times.

Suicide is even more frequent among older people. The highest rates are found in men over 50. Before the American Foundation for Suicide Prevention (AFSP) was formed, there was no national not-for-profit organization dedicated to funding the research, education, and treatment programs necessary to prevent suicide. Over the past 20 years, AFSP has changed that.

The primary focus of AFSP is suicide prevention. They accomplish their goals through research and education and through reaching out both to people with mood **disorders** and to those affected by suicide. To fully achieve its mission, AFSP engages in the following strategies:

- Provides funding for academic scholars to conduct research

- Offers educational programs for professionals such as hospital staff and school counselors

- Educates the public about mood disorders and suicide prevention through videos and print materials

- Promotes policies and legislation that affect suicide and prevention such as gun control

- Provides programs and resources for survivors of suicide loss and involves them in the work of the foundation, such as helping to raise funds through walkathons and educating other survivors on managing the healing process

TEEN SUICIDE PREVENTION CAMPAIGN

"Suicide Shouldn't Be a Secret" is the key theme of the American Foundation for Suicide Prevention's youth suicide prevention campaign. They have produced a noncommercial broadcast for radio and television known as a public service announcement to educate the public about suicide among teenagers. This public service announcement tells teens that they should never keep the secret of a friend who says he or she wants to kill him or herself. They should always tell an adult, counselor, or parent. It is always better to lose a friendship and save a life! The public service announcements feature actual teenagers who have had a suicidal friend or have lost a friend to suicide. They tell teens how to recognize the warning signs when a friend is in a suicidal crisis.

According to AFSP, the five major warning signs of suicide are as follows:

- feelings of sadness or hopelessness, often accompanied by anxiety

- declining school performance or no longer doing well in school

- loss of pleasure/interest in social and sports activities

- sleeping too little or too much

- change in weight or appetite

If you have a friend who has at least three of these warning signs, you can take action. AFSP recommends these three steps:

- Take your friend's actions seriously.

- Encourage your friend to seek professional help, accompany if necessary.

- Talk to an adult you trust. Don't be alone in helping your friend.

AFSP reports that depression is a common and real illness that interferes with a student's ability to be productive and enjoy friends, family, sports, or school. Suicide is currently the third leading cause of death. Remember, if you have a friend in crisis–tell someone!

Walkathons for fund-raising

Out of the Darkness Overnight is a fund-raising walk where millions of people who either lost someone to suicide or are interested in the fight against suicide join together to walk when the sun sets and continue walking until sunrise the next day. These walkathons make a statement that AFSP can and must take steps to bring suicide and mood disorders out of the darkness.

THE RESEARCH

AFSP is exclusively dedicated to understanding and preventing suicide through research and education and to reaching out to people with mental disorders and families who lost someone to suicide. The

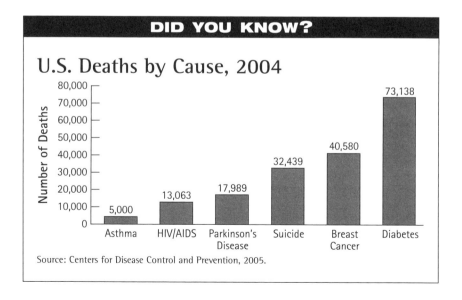

DID YOU KNOW?

U.S. Deaths by Cause, 2004

Source: Centers for Disease Control and Prevention, 2005.

amount of money spent on research to study the causes of suicide is much less than the amount spent on other causes of death, such as breast cancer. While it is very important to study all causes of death, U.S. families lost 32,439 people to suicide in 2004; there were 13,063 deaths caused by HIV/AIDS in the same year. Despite this fact, more money is spent on HIV/AIDS research than on suicide research.

AFSP faces many challenges in suicide research because suicide is not a single "illness" but a fatal result of various disorders such as depression, **bipolar disorder, schizophrenia, anxiety disorder,** alcoholism and other substance abuse, **adjustment disorder, conduct disorder,** and personality traits such as impulsivity and aggression. All of these disorders can cause suicidal behavior. If these disorders are present, however, it does not mean the person will become suicidal but only that there is a possibility that suicidal behavior could develop.

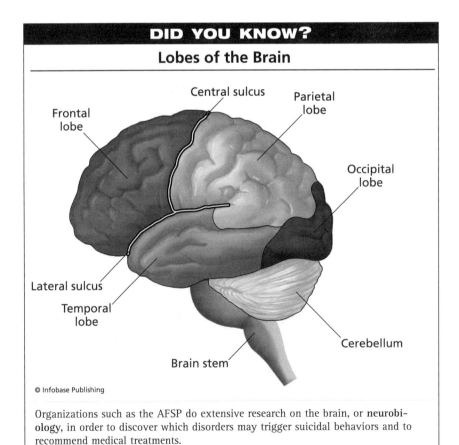

DID YOU KNOW?

Lobes of the Brain

Central sulcus

Parietal lobe

Frontal lobe

Occipital lobe

Lateral sulcus

Temporal lobe

Cerebellum

Brain stem

© Infobase Publishing

Organizations such as the AFSP do extensive research on the brain, or **neurobiology,** in order to discover which disorders may trigger suicidal behaviors and to recommend medical treatments.

Source: American Foundation for Suicide Prevention

DID YOU KNOW?

Highest Suicide Rate in the World

	Suicide Rate (per 100,000 people)	Year
Lithuania	70.1	2004
Belarus	63.3	2003
Russian Federation	61.6	2004
Kazakhstan	51.0	2003
Hungary	44.9	2003

For most of the 1990s, Hungary had the highest suicide rate in the world. As of 2007, Lithuania took over that position. It is suggested that the high rate in these regions is the result of political unrest due to the change from communism in some states and the high unemployment rate.

Source: World Health Organization, 2007.

Therefore, research on suicidal behavior becomes extremely important so that the general population can be made aware which mental disorders are more likely to contribute to suicidal thoughts, attempts, and completions—and what can be done to control the risk of suicide if a mental disorder is present.

AFSP plays an active role in seeking to reduce suicide rates through participating in projects to develop, implement, and evaluate approaches to suicide prevention. In its suicide prevention projects, AFSP partners with individuals, organizations, and institutions throughout the United States and abroad who share their dedication to finding new and better ways to prevent suicide. A key goal of each project is to distribute information about what has been learned through articles that reach the general audience and mental health workers.

See also: Suicide Prevention

FURTHER READING

Alt, Jeff. *A Hike for Mike: An Uplifting Adventure Across the Sierra Nevada for Depression Awareness.* Cincinnati, Ohio: Dreams Shared Publications, 2005.

Henden, John. *Preventing Suicide: The Solution Focused Approach.* New York: Wiley, 2008.

Nelson, Richard E., Ph.D., and Judith C. Galas. *The Power to Prevent Suicide: A Guide for Teens Helping Teens.* Minneapolis, Minn.: Free Spirit Publishing, 1994.

■ BIOLOGY OF SUICIDAL BEHAVIOR

The biological, or physical, predisposition toward suicide, the act of taking one's own life, which involves mental **disorders** that can lead to suicide. Ninety percent or more of completed suicides are due to some form of mental instability that is often associated with biological changes. Chemical imbalances in the brain are one example of the biological change that can take place. These are generally what cause individuals to have distorted thoughts about ending their lives. There are three chemicals in the brain that affect mood:

- serotonin
- norepinephrine
- dopamine

The first and most talked about chemical is **serotonin**. Serotonin is a **neurotransmitter** in the brain or central nervous system that has a major influence over several brain functions. Most studies indicate that impulsivity and aggressive behavior are related to lower levels of serotonin in the brain. This chemical is also linked to such things as appetite, sleep, mood behavior, and **depression**. The linkage of serotonin to depression is a result of decreased levels of serotonin in the brain. Medications that can enhance serotonin levels in the brain are helpful in treating the depression that can lead to suicidal behavior. Studies show that those who suffer from clinical depression due to a **chemical deficiency,** such as low levels of serotonin and are not being treated by a **medication** that raises the serotonin levels, such as a **serotonin reuptake inhibitor (SSRI),** have a 15 percent chance of suicide among those suffering from major depressive disorder due to a chemical imbalance.

Everyone has a physiological stress structure within them that affects the chemical functions of the brain. When the body is not capable of physically handling **stressors** or stress buildup, its coping mechanisms weaken. When we experience stress, our adrenal glands produce the hormones norepinephrine and epinephrine, or "noradrenaline" and "adrenaline." Norepinephrine is released when a host of physiological changes are activated by a stressful event. This chemical gives the body

Neurotransmitters and the Brain

Neurotransmitter	Functions in the brain
Serotonin	Regulates emotion, anxiety, agitation, and gastrointestinal function
Norepinephrine	Regulates emotion and attention
Dopamine	Regulates movement and pleasure

When one or more of the chemicals listed in the left column changes, so do mood and behavior, sometimes leading to suicide.

resources in order to meet the stressful challenges. When there is not enough norepinephrine in the body, the coping mechanisms can break down, which sometimes result in suicidal thoughts.

A third chemical that affects mood is **dopamine**. When dopamine is released, it provides feelings of enjoyment and allows us to stay motivated to do, or continue doing, certain activities. Dopamine is released by naturally rewarding experiences such as eating food or touching, like getting a good hug from a family member or friend. This preprogrammed reward system makes sure that people eat, desire to comfort one another, and basically survive. Without enough dopamine, people feel the opposite of enjoyment and motivation—they feel fatigued and depressed and experience a lack of drive and motivation.

Experts in the psychiatric field claim that 90 percent or more of suicides are due to some form of mental disorder that is often associated with biological changes. The neurobiological changes can consist of predisposing personality traits such as impulsivity and aggressive behavior, as well as external forces such as the impact of trauma, substance abuse, and chronic stress.

Q & A

Question: Why do depressive illnesses sometimes lead to suicidal thoughts?

Answer: There is a direct link between depressive illnesses and suicide. The number one cause of suicide is untreated depression.

Depressive illnesses can distort thinking, so a person can have trouble thinking clearly or rationally. They may not know they have a treatable illness, or they may think they can't be helped. Their illness can cause thoughts of hopelessness and helplessness, which may then lead to suicidal thoughts. They just can't see any other way out. That's why it is so important to educate people on the symptoms of depression and other depressive illnesses and on the warning signs of suicide, so that people suffering from these illnesses can get the help they need. People must understand that depression and other related depressive illnesses are treatable and that they can feel better.

TREATMENT FOR CHEMICAL IMBALANCES

There is medication to increase the levels of these chemicals—antidepressants. The drugs function by slowing down the process that breaks down neurotransmitters in the brain. Neurotransmitters are necessary in the brain in order to send out nerve impulses across the synapse, moving the signal from one brain cell to another. The idea behind treatment with the antidepressants is that as a result of its action, increased levels of neurotransmitters build up in the central nervous system and help individuals come out of a depressed state. These medicines may take a few weeks to work through the system and become effective, but they work well and are generally safe.

There are three main groups of antidepressants: selective serotonin reuptake inhibitors (SSRIs), tricyclics (TCAs), and monoamine oxidase inhibitors (MAOIs). SSRIs such as the prescription drug Lexapro are the newest class of antidepressants. They help to relieve the symptoms of depression by increasing the available supply of serotonin.

Another new class of antidepressants is the selective serotonin and norepinephrine reuptake inhibitors (SNRIs). This medication affects both norepinephrine and serotonin levels in the brain. While low levels of both neurotransmitters are associated with depression, norepinephrine is thought to be involved more with alertness and energy, while serotonin influences mood. By increasing levels of both, SNRIs work on different aspects of depression. Reduction of depression in a patient is a doctor's main goal.

According to Dr. Jeffrey Kelsey, medical director at Georgia Institute of Mood and Anxiety Disorders, all of the antidepressants that are available in the U.S. market today are equally effective when it comes to response rates. Dr. Kelsey explains that when it comes to reduction in depression, however, the data shows that SNRIs, dual-acting antidepressants, will in some patients present an advantage. However, many doctors don't know which patients will benefit from one approach over the other and have to go by trial and error. This is why it is important to comply with the doctor's wishes and stay in touch with the doctor if any changes occur in your body or in your mental behavior.

GENETIC FACTORS

The genetic components that influence a person's tendency to complete or attempt suicide can be seen in a **family history** of suicide, aggressiveness, impulsivity, and chronic substance abuse. There are two genetic sources accountable for increased risk of suicide: (1) a genetic liability to mental illness, and (2) a genetic liability to impulsive aggression. When both come together, the risk for suicide is high.

Other factors that are not genetic can also cause a predisposition to suicide. These include social factors like isolation, childhood abuse, sexual assault, and the early death of a parent. Social factors in many cases are independent of genetic factors.

CHANGES IN THE BIOLOGY OF THE BRAIN

The frontal lobe of the brain is where the memory sensors are located. How you think, communicate, feel, plan, and carry out a certain task is all wrapped up in memory. A depressed person has the inability to retrieve positive happy memories and can only retrieve sad and negative memories. It is this section of the brain that contains most of the dopamine-sensitive **neurons.** The dopamine system is associated with pleasure, long-term memory, planning, and drive. A low level of dopamine in the brain is associated with depression. Another important fact is that the front lobe of the brain is not fully developed until age 25, according the National Institute of Mental Health. Teenagers who abuse **drugs** are interfering with the development of the brain, which could lead to permanent damage. Damage to the frontal lobe can causes mood changes associated with various mental disorders such as serious depression and **schizophrenia.**

Many American teens who report experiencing weeks of hopelessness and loss of interest in normal daily activities are using marijuana and other drugs, making their situation worse, according to a White House report released in May 2008. The report from the White House Office of National Drug Control Policy (ONDCP) reveals that marijuana use can worsen depression and lead to more serious mental disorders, such as schizophrenia, anxiety, and even suicide. Suicide victims appear to have overactivity in certain parts of the brain or imbalanced levels of chemicals that affect how stress is handled.

Many researchers have found that biological changes within the brain, such as chemical imbalances, can be caused by severe childhood trauma. Childhood trauma generates immediate biological, psychological, and behavioral effects, some of which can last for long periods of time. When the brain is still developing, exposure to trauma can cause significant changes in the anatomy and physiology of the development of the brain and can delay certain functions such as motor skills, sensory skills, or how one thinks and figures things out. This is because the human brain is not a finished organ at birth; it takes another 10 to 20 years for the development of the brain to be completed. If the brain is unable to mature properly due to childhood trauma, psychosocial and behavior consequences can develop. For instance, a child can develop low self-esteem or abuse substances as well as engage in delinquent behavior—all pathways to suicidal behavior.

TEENS SPEAK

What Do I Have to Live For?

We had just moved from one house to another in Karmah, Iraq. Luckily, we had the good fortune of not being shot at or having a roadside bomb go off on our vehicles this time. As we got closer to our destination, we turned on all our lights and pulled our night vision goggles off. We saw the family scamper off in the distance with bundles on their backs. It made no difference for me. I had mail! I could not wait to open up the perfume scented piece of America that my girlfriend had sent me. It had been a month since I had a shower. About three weeks since I had changed my clothes. Any brief respite from the dreariness of my life at this point would make me happier.

When we had secured the house I sat in a room alone so I could read the letter and just enjoy this piece of Americana that made me not hate my life. As I impatiently opened up the letter, I read each word carefully. I needed to be connected to her in some way and this was the best I could do. As I was reading, a light switch clicked in my head. She was breaking up with me. The love of my life is leaving me. As I set the letter down, I looked at the pictures she had sent me earlier months in my deployment. Happy. In love. Together. Now none of that mattered.

As I walked outside, I chambered a round into the assault rifle I carried. I hate my life. I have nothing to live for. I don't feel like living every day like I'm going to die. The fear of being shot, being blown up, being killed for someone else's war. What the hell am I doing here? All this ran through my mind as I sat down and put the barrel of the rifle in my mouth and closed my eyes. I put the weapon on 3 round burst. No need to screw this up like I screwed up my relationships. I slowly eased the slack from the trigger and waited for the nothingness.

The coward's way out. I'm better than this. I've seen my friends get blown up, I've been shot at, I've seen everything that no one who is 19 should see, but as history tells us they always do. I slowly eased my finger off the trigger. What would the rest of my platoon members think? Coward. That's all I would ever be to them if I pulled the trigger. All the praise over my speed and abilities in my job would be all for nothing. I would be one step below deserters. I sat and silently reflected on life right there on top of a dirty blanket used for dry dates. I have so much more to live for. I'm young.

Q & A

Question: Do certain antidepressants such as Prozac, Zoloft, and Paxil cause more suicides among teenagers?

Answer: The U.S. Food and Drug Administration put a warning on most antidepressants that reads like this:

Suicidality in Children and Adolescents

Antidepressants increase the risk of suicidal thinking and behavior (suicidality) in children and adolescents with major depressive disorder (MDD) and other psychiatric disorders. Anyone considering the use of [*Drug Name*] or any other antidepressant in a child or adolescent must balance this risk with the clinical need. Patients who are started on therapy should be observed closely for clinical worsening, suicidality, or unusual changes in behavior. Families and caregivers should be advised of the need for close observation and communication with the prescriber. [*Drug Name*] is not approved for use in pediatric patients except for patients with [*Any approved pediatric claims here*].

The drugs that must carry this warning include:

- Anafranil (clomipramine HCl)
- Aventyl (nortriptyline HCl)
- Celexa (citalopram HBr)
- Cymbalta (duloxetine HCl)
- Desyrel (trazodone HCl)
- Effexor (venlafaxine HCl)
- Elavil (amitriptyline HCl)
- Lexapro (escitalopram oxalate)
- Limbitrol (chlordiazepoxide/amitriptyline)
- Ludiomil (maprotiline HCl)
- Luvox (fluvoxamine maleate)
- Marplan (isocarboxazid)
- Nardil (phenelzine sulfate)
- Nefazodone HCl
- Norpramin (desipramine HCl)
- Pamelor (nortriptyline HCl)
- Parnate (tranylcypromine sulfate)
- Paxil (paroxetine HCl)
- Pexeva (paroxetine mesylate)
- Prozac (fluoxetine HCl)
- Remeron (mirtazapine)
- Sarafem (fluoxetine HCl)
- Sinequan (doxepin HCl)
- Surmontil (trimipramine)
- Symbyax (olanzapine/fluoxetine)
- Tofranil (imipramine HCl)
- Tofranil-PM (impiramine pamoate)
- Triavil (perphenaine/amitriptyline)
- Vivactil (protriptyline HCl)

- Wellbutrin (bupropion HCl)
- Zoloft (sertraline HCl)
- Zyban (bupropion HCl)

What this warning indicates is that these drugs could cause suicidality or suicidal thinking because of the reaction an individual may have to the medication. However, the taking of these medications needs to be monitored and watched closely; they do not directly cause someone to complete suicide. Most psychiatrists strongly believe that the risk of suicide is much higher in a depressed person who does not receive treatment than is any risk caused by these medications.

See also: Culture and Suicide; Gender and Suicide

FURTHER READING
Haley, James, ed., *Death & Dying* (Opposing Viewpoints Series). Farmington Hills, Mich.: Greenhaven Press, 2002.
Henden, John. *Preventing Suicide: The Solution Focused Approach.* New York: Wiley, 2008.
Lezine, De Quincy, and David Brent. *Eight Stories Up: An Adolescent Chooses Hope over Suicide.* New York: Oxford University Press, 2008.
Maris, Ronald W. *Biology of Suicide.* New York: Guildford Press, 1986.

■ CLUSTER SUICIDES

A group of suicides that occur in the same community, region, or social network, over a period of days or months, usually not more than 60 to 90 days, although sometimes longer. In 1983, for example, five teenagers in Plano, Texas, killed themselves in less than six weeks. In that same year, 15 others attempted suicide.

According to the Centers for Disease Control and Prevention (CDC), five teenagers kill themselves in the United States every day. Therefore, when there are five suicides in one community in a short period—especially within weeks—it is alarming, particularly if the teens knew one another. A **double suicide** occurs when a couple or two friends commit suicide. In a cluster suicide, however, the victims do not always know one another but may be connected in some other way. They may have had some knowledge of the other suicides through their community or a social network, which can be anything from friends hanging around in the same crowd to being members of the same club or organization to going to the same school.

CAUSES OF CLUSTER SUICIDE

Cluster suicide—also referred to as contagion, copycat, or imitation suicide—is additionally defined as a suicide that creates a stimulus or incentive for other suicides within a given community and that is caused by the stimulus. In other words, cluster suicide is a process in which being exposed to the suicide of one person can influence others to take their own lives.

Suicide contagion differs slightly. The suicide that may be considered contagious (perhaps because it is an idolized celebrity) is not confined to suicides occurring in one geographic area. However, the influence comes, instead, from the media such as newspaper reports or live television reports and affects the whole nation. Studies have shown that mass media coverage such as newspaper articles and television reports along with fictional dramatizations have led to a higher rate of suicides during a specified time period after the media exposure. That time period is usually very close to the date of the suicide being exposed over the media.

Suicide contagion, therefore, is a process in which suicidal behavior is imitated by one or more individuals, following the awareness of a recent suicide threat, attempt, completion, or fictional depiction of such behavior. For example, after the suicide death of rock star Kurt Cobain in April 1994, many suicide prevention specialists worried about imitations and copycat suicides. Cobain had many fans of his grunge band Nirvana, and some fans may have been vulnerable or predisposed to suicide and thus influenced by his behavior.

Reporting a suicide over the media can have some benefits such as emphasizing the need to develop community efforts to prevent suicide, explaining how to identify persons at high risk for suicide, or identifying where to go for help. Glorification or memorialization of the suicide victim, however, in a way that suggests that society is honoring the suicidal behavior can be hazardous. At that point, vulnerable persons may mistakenly perceive suicide as an attractive solution to their problems.

Q & A

Question: Do people really commit copycat suicides?

Answer: Yes, there is evidence to show that copycat suicides do occur under some circumstances. If someone is already vulnerable (depressed, showing some warning signs, has made a previous attempt), one suicide can be a **trigger** to another. This is especially pronounced in youth. Conditions that can increase the risk of copycat suicides include high-profile celebrities, sensational portrayals of suicide in the media, or inadvertent glorification of a suicide victim. These factors have the unintended effect of portraying suicide as a viable option.

FAMOUS CASES

In 1997, South Boston, Massachusetts, was the site of a string of completed suicides and attempts. Six young males hanged themselves in a span of seven months. What was clear in South Boston was that there were a lot of individuals in the community who lost hope and were very unhappy because the neighborhood became contaminated with **drugs,** drug abusers, broken homes, and high school dropouts who could not find jobs. The misery and sadness left young kids in the streets with no commitments, too much unstructured time, and no idea what to do next. Many had no real direction and felt misunderstood. In that same year, 1997, there were nearly 70 teenagers hospitalized for attempts or thoughts of suicide, most of them males.

According to the *American Journal of Public Health,* more than 4,500 young adults under the age of 24 kill themselves each year. Anywhere from 45 to more than 200 of those suicides, or 1 to 5 percent, occur in clusters. Generally, the youth who take their own lives after being exposed to a suicide are already vulnerable and at risk for suicide. In 2000, there were four suicides in a six-month period in a suburb of Texas near Austin. The victims attended the same small and financially exclusive school. All of the victims were diagnosed with various forms of **depression** or showed signs of depression. Three of the deceased were receiving psychiatric and psychological services at the time; another had a history of receiving counseling. Each youth was receiving one or more prescribed **medications** as part of the treatment regimen, and all were using illicit drugs.

The suicide that stimulated the cluster had occurred eight months before the other suicides. This victim had jumped to his death in

October 1999. The first cluster victim hanged himself that following June 2000; the second victim hanged himself in August; the third victim hanged himself in October; and the fourth victim hanged himself in November. All four of the victims used the same method of death—asphyxiation (to become unconscious by inadequate oxygen or inability to breathe). Because of the many similarities, there is a strong contagion connection between each suicide. The suicidal act was reinforced by imitating the chosen method of hanging. One suicide used the belt owned by the suicide victim just before him and given to him by the victim's mother.

Q & A

Question: My best friend's father killed himself. Does this mean that my friend may kill himself too? Is it contagious?

Answer: Just because your friend's father took his own life does not mean your friend will take his own life. However, this is a very complex question to answer because there are many factors involved that could make your friend predisposed to complete suicide. For example, if the father suffered from depression or some other mental **disorder** and the mental disorder played a major factor in the suicide, there is a possibility that your friend could inherit the mental disorder. It is the mental disorder that can be "catching" or genetic, and this could put your friend at risk. Your friend also might model his father's behavior when he feels totally overwhelmed and cannot cope. Many teenagers think of suicide but never, ever act upon it. In your friend's case, he may think about suicide and go further because his father did.

Finally, a suicide in the family puts most of the members at risk for suicide. Feelings of anger, guilt, fear, and sadness are natural responses to a loved one's suicide. These complex emotions make it difficult to get through the grieving process. If your friend has difficulty grieving and is not allowed to mourn his father openly—or if he is suffering from an unusual amount of guilt—he needs help. All things considered, your friend should be given as much love and understanding as possible. Don't be afraid to offer to help him or to get him help from a school counselor, respected adviser, or religious leader.

Fact Or Fiction?

Suicide rates are highest among African-American females.

The Facts: Black females have the lowest rate of suicide among both males and females. There is little known of any suicide clusters among African-Americans and especially among African-American females. Studies have indicated that females of all ethnic backgrounds have lower rates of completed suicides and higher rates of suicide attempts than males. The same is for black females—low completed suicides and higher attempts than African-American males.

PREVENTION

Because of clustering, when a report comes over the news of the suicide of a well-known celebrity, prevention specialists become highly concerned and are on high alert to watch over any young adult who may be vulnerable to suicide. If a school friend takes his or her own life, it is a time for all students to come together and protect one another against the pain and anguish caused by a suicide. Talk to teachers, counselors, advisers, or anyone who will listen about how you feel because of the suicide.

Stay in groups and do not isolate yourself. Engage in group activities such as ice-skating or roller skating; go to the library with friends; have sleepovers; and stay together as much as possible for the first six weeks or more following the event. If friends of the suicide victim feel suicidal, let them talk about it openly, and be sure to bring them to an adult or tell an adult. It is normal to feel mentally "sick" after a suicide in your school. It may make you feel sad, guilty, angry, and helpless. Seek help as soon as possible.

See also: Cults and Suicide; Media Coverage

FURTHER READING

Cobain, Beverly, and Jean Larch. *Dying to Be Free: A Healing Guide for Families After a Suicide.* Center City, Minn.: Hazelden, 2006.

Joiner, Thomas. *Why People Die by Suicide.* Cambridge, Mass.: Harvard University Press, 2005.

■ COPYCAT SUICIDES
See: Cluster Suicides

■ COUNSELING
See: Therapies and Psychodynamics

■ CULTS AND SUICIDE
An interrelated, unified group devoted to certain beliefs that tend to be different from mainstream beliefs and practices, sometimes involving ritual suicide. Religious cults whose members believe that life is better after death often become "death cults." Cult members often see group or **mass suicides** as a release.

On November 18, 1978, more than 900 people died by their own hand in Jonestown, a settlement northwest of Guyana, named after its creator, Jim Jones. He had formed a religious organization called the Peoples Temple, which originated out of Indiana and, later, California. He eventually moved his congregation to Guyana (located on the northern coast of South America) to form a commune to be inhabited by members of the Peoples Temple. The member's belief that life would be better separated from family, friends, and the rest of the world controlled their thinking, actions, and feelings. Jim Jones was able to pressure his members to drink poison and kill themselves. People often wonder how others could join such a cult, and they wish to know why cult members would kill themselves just because they were told to.

It starts with an individual having feelings of alienation or **depression.** When people feel alienated, they experience the self as alien or not fitting in. They are engulfed with negative feelings all the time, while people around them seem able to feel good, have fun with one another, and feel secure. Persons feeling alienated feel separate from those warm feelings. They have negative feelings all the time, as if a black cloud were hanging overhead. Oftentimes these feelings are coupled with a sense that they are being drawn to destructive behavior. When teenagers feel that they do not fit in, they tend to look for those who feel the same way and find "bad company." They may become a part of a delinquent group of people who have the same negative feelings and who feel alienated from everyone else. Teenagers who feel alienated from everyone else will sometimes join a cult or a church of devil worshippers. The following is a testimonial:

> This feeling of detachment, separation, aloneness is not new for me. I suppose I became aware of this feeling in jr. high when cliques were in abundance. Not only did I not understand cliques, but I was torn by having to choose friendships according to who was in what clique. This was extremely stressful and emotionally distressing to me, and the cliques continued through high school. I never felt like I "fit" anywhere during this time period.

> To this day, I continue to feel this lack of connection with many people, especially in a group of people that already have established, close friendships. I suppose I feel like an unwelcomed intruder in these social situations.

Feelings such as these can develop into forms of self-injury or self-destructive behaviors. Suicidal gestures such as attempts or near-fatal car accidents are high among this group of teenagers and young adults.

REASONS FOR JOINING A CULT

Feelings of alienation can move individuals toward joining a cult. However, they must identify or feel a connection to the group. If a connection is generated, an individual may want to become a part of a group and join to develop a feeling of belonging. Some researchers believe that there is a strong sense for fulfillment of psychological needs—conscious or subconscious. Some alienated individuals also join because they seek psychological manipulation, which occurs when one allows the leader to influence your thoughts and control your thoughts. They want to be led.

Cults known for their mass or group suicides in which all members agree to commit suicide together are also known for giving their members unconditional love and acceptance as well as a new identity based on the group. Ultimately, members are controlled. And as previously mentioned, individuals who feel alienated by the people around them will often join these cults to feel a sense of belonging. They become dedicated to some person or leader.

Heaven's Gate

In 1997, 38 cult members and their religious leader were found dead in a house located in an upscale neighborhood in San Diego, California. Their deaths occurred on the same evening that a comet called Hale-Bopp appeared in the sky. Heaven's Gate was the name of this religious group, founded in the United States by Marshall Applewhite. The group suicide was completed after Applewhite convinced 38 followers to take their own lives so that their souls could take a ride on a spaceship that they believed was hiding behind the comet. They also believed that the Earth was about to be wiped clean and that their only chance to survive was to leave the Earth immediately.

Developing their belief system from the Bible's Book of Revelation, the founders of Heaven's Gate believed that a human being could completely transform through hard work, a strict diet, fasting, and practicing great discipline by abstaining from alcohol, tobacco, sex, and most material possessions. In preparing to kill themselves, they wanted to make certain that their bodies were cleansed of any impurities and drank citrus juices ritually.

Fact Or Fiction?

After joining a cult, leaving the cult can become as traumatic as the death of a loved one.

The Facts: Two Harvard Medical School psychiatrists wrote an article based on their experience of treating former members of cults who were reentering society and trying to get back into normal life. They found that their clients were having a difficult experience, and the doctors compared the situation of former members of cults to that of ex-prisoners, soldiers returning from war, and those emerging from divorce or death of a spouse. Although the term for this experience—*post-cult trauma*—is a term that is often disputed, many scholars acknowledge that abandoning a cult can be extremely traumatic for some, yet not for all.

HOW CULTS FIND VICTIMS

The following is a true story of one teenager's deadly encounter with a cult. Sammy Bloom's story is told by his mother, Lois Bloom.

TEEN'S MOM SPEAKS

Sammy's Story

Piecing together the few clues [our son] Sammy left behind, we discovered he left with three strangers who were part of a religious cult. Investigating the group, we were told it was a very destructive group that used hypnosis and brainwashing techniques based on those used on U.S. soldiers by North Korea. The result of hypnosis and brainwashing techniques causes a shift in personality or "depersonalization." Former members reported the drug Phencyclidine (PCP or Angel Dust) was used to seduce new members to join. The drug was used to induce dissociative behavior in order to instill post-hypnotic suggestions that can create a complete behavior change. The cult admits to using marijuana, which they call a natural herb.

Quickly our family put together a plan to look for Sammy with our family and friends. We searched intensely for the entire 17 days he was missing but never found him. On the 17th-day, Sammy called us from Roma, Texas. He wanted to come home.

The morning he disappeared, Sammy attended classes and was driving home for lunch when he saw three hitchhikers wearing Christ-like clothes along the side of the road. Intrigued, he stopped and asked them if they were in a play at college. They said they'd tell him about themselves if he took them home for lunch.

Within hours Sammy had withdrawn all the money from his checking and savings accounts, sold his prized vintage golf clubs, gave them all the money, and left with them, taking only a toothbrush and quilt which he used as a sleeping bag. . . . Sammy's next 17 days were intense and difficult. He was brainwashed, intimidated, deceived, condemned, became mesmerized, and rapidly lost his capability for independent thought. During Sammy's indoctrination, his life was totally controlled by the cult members. They monitored his food and liquid intake, limited his sleep, told him when to go to the restroom and had him smoking cigarettes that they rolled for him (Sammy had always been a non-smoker). Told that God provides, they begged for food and ate from dumpsters. . . . Wearing Christ-like clothes made of white sheets and walking bare-footed, Sammy walked and hitchhiked to Texas with them.

When Sammy's painful feet became unbearable to walk on because of blisters and stones that were embedded in them, he asked the cult members for help. Getting none, he told them he couldn't walk any further. Screaming at Sammy, they told him that if he didn't stay with them that he and his family would burn in Hell. Sammy left them anyway. When he left the group he really thought he could bring all of our family into the group.

. . . During the first week, we hired two different exit counselors to have Sammy deprogrammed, believing it was a legitimate process for freeing Sammy's mind to get him back to thinking rationally. . . . The deprogramming did not work. Shortly after, Sammy became very suicidal, making several suicidal threats and gestures. We took him to the UCLA Neuro-Psychiatric Institute (NPI) for evaluation. The psychologist evaluating Sammy said he was in a "reactive psychosis," was highly suicidal, and needed to be hospitalized immediately. He was hospitalized at UCLA. While giving them family history, we told them my father had bipolar disorder most of his life. Treatment for Sammy was extremely difficult because of the severe reactions he had from medications. In addition to psychosis, Sammy became depressed; he stopped eating and talking and was on "suicide watch."

As a last resort, the doctors gave Sammy electro-convulsive therapy (ECT). The treatments (he had a total of nine ECT treatments) were immediately successful, and the doctors stabilized his medication and continued to treat him with psychotherapy. While at NPI, Louis J. West, M.D. . . . oversaw the treatment given Sammy. Dr. West told us Sammy was on the verge of a psychotic episode when recruited by the cult, and because of the severity of his brainwashing experience had a much more severe psychotic episode. Sammy was hospitalized for three months.

Eventually, Sammy killed himself, leaving behind a note to his family that still showed signs of his indoctrination with the cult. His belief that he could bring his family into the cult remained. Among other things, he wrote, "Please obey God's laws, No Killing, No Sex, and No Materialism." Never having known anyone who had a cult experience, it was not something we ever thought to discuss with our children. Now we believe that all families should discuss the danger of cults with their teenagers before they move from home. It's an experience that could happen to any one, but we have learned lonely, idealistic, impressionable college students are especially vulnerable.

Unfortunately, Sammy's psychotic episode would not have been as severe had he not had the intense experience of being brainwashed. Dr. West said Sammy could never be fully deprogrammed because the cult ideology and his psychotic experience were mixed together in his mind. It's alarming how many mentally ill persons have been victimized by cults. We have known of several who have killed themselves.

AFTERTHOUGHTS: When Sammy met the cult members, he was more vulnerable to being recruited by a cult because of the numerous changes in his life. He was living in new circumstances, had the loss of a girl he was in love with, lost friends due to his recent move, had the loss of his golfing buddies that he saw every day when he was playing golf for years, and the loss of his dream of playing with the golf team (he had counted on continuing to play throughout his college years). Furthermore, Sammy was idealistic, inquisitive, trusting, and naïve.

Furthermore, Dr. West believed Sammy was probably experiencing the onset of a serious mental illness shortly before he met the three strangers. It is widely known that those who are searching for a new direction in their lives are more vulnerable to cult recruitment. The cult offered Sammy instant, simplistic solutions to his problems. Moreover, Sammy was "duped," the process, a seduction was not a mutually beneficial agreement. Dr. Eli Shapiro of Boston University Medical Center describes today's destructive cults as using "menticide," a dangerous form of mental coercion in which the free mind is attacked by Pavlovian conditioning techniques, without the victim's conscious knowledge or consent. Experts say that all people are potentially vulnerable at different times in their lives. It is thought that cults use a systematic program of psychological manipulation to convince people to join them and remain in them.

Sammy's story is not unique. Unfortunately, many adolescents and young adults are recruited into these types of religious groups. There are between 3,000 and 5,000 professed cults that exist in the United States, and most of them are not widely known and do not engage in violent, criminal acts.

See also: Cluster Suicides; Media Coverage: Suicide Prevention

FURTHER READING

Bromley, David, and J. Gordon Melton. *Cults, Religion and Violence.* Cambridge: Cambridge University Press, 2002.

Singer, M., and J. Lalich. *Cults in our Midst: The Continuing Fight Against Their Hidden Menace.* Hoboken, N.J.: Jossey-Bass, 1995.

■ CULTURE AND SUICIDE

The values, beliefs, behaviors, and material things that together form a way of life for a population or group of people and the effect of that way of life on a society's suicide rate. Culture includes what we think, how we act, and what we own. Different groups of people have higher rates of suicide than other groups. For example, men complete suicide at higher rates than women; people who live in Montana have higher rates of suicide than people who live in New Jersey; people who live in Belarus—a country in eastern Europe—have higher rates of suicide than those who live in the United States. What constitutes these differences? Why do boys complete suicide more than girls?

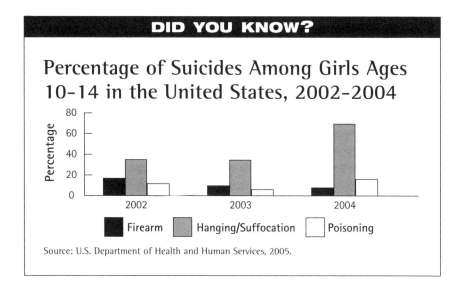

Percentage of Suicides Among Girls Ages 10-14 in the United States, 2002-2004

Source: U.S. Department of Health and Human Services, 2005.

GENDER DIFFERENCES

According to the World Health Organization (WHO), in 2001, males in western nations completed suicide at much higher rates than females. However, in China, females completed suicide more than males.

In the United States, there are more than 30,000 suicides a year. More than 24,000 of those suicides are males. There are also more than 250,000 attempts that are reported each year, and the majority of those attempts are made by females. Thus, males complete more suicides, and females attempt more. One of the obvious reasons for the difference in suicide rates is that boys use a more lethal means, such as a gun, while females may take pills or cut themselves. Experts are finding that females are beginning to use more lethal means such as hanging. Another reason for the difference is that males may also be abusing **drugs** or alcohol while they are in suicidal crisis, and therefore they are less able to control an urge of suicide. More than 60 percent of those who commit suicide or attempt suicide are generally suffering from some form of **depression.** Males are less willing than females to seek counseling, stay in counseling, or comply with any form of treatment that may be needed if in counseling. Untreated depression is one of the major causes of suicide.

DID YOU KNOW?

Suicides by State, 2005

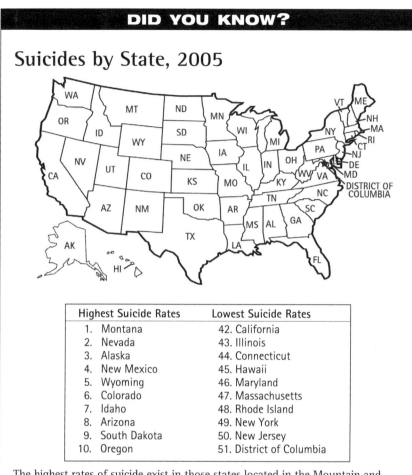

Highest Suicide Rates	Lowest Suicide Rates
1. Montana	42. California
2. Nevada	43. Illinois
3. Alaska	44. Connecticut
4. New Mexico	45. Hawaii
5. Wyoming	46. Maryland
6. Colorado	47. Massachusetts
7. Idaho	48. Rhode Island
8. Arizona	49. New York
9. South Dakota	50. New Jersey
10. Oregon	51. District of Columbia

The highest rates of suicide exist in those states located in the Mountain and Central Regions of the United States.

Source: The American Foundation for Suicide Prevention, 2005.

REGIONAL DIFFERENCES

Suicide rates are higher in Montana and Wyoming than they are in New York and New Jersey. What do you suppose goes on in the Mountain regions that is not happening in the Eastern part of the country? One theory is that there are more hunting guns in the homes of those in the Mountain and Central parts of the United States. Guns are the leading method of suicide for males, and if every home has one, then that creates a problem. Another theory is that there is less access to hospitals and emergency rooms in that part of the country, whereas on the East Coast there are emergency rooms and hospitals less than a mile apart in many cities. In rural areas, hospitals may be hundreds of miles apart. Suicides also vary among countries.

IMMIGRANTS

According to the *Washington Post,* the United States accepts more legal immigrants as permanent residents than any other country in the world. The number of immigrants in the United States totals approximately 40 million or more, and that number is only the ones that can be counted legally. When a foreign-born individual or family moves to this country, there are factors that can put them at risk for suicide. For instance, the problems and challenges of trying to adjust

DID YOU KNOW?

Highest Suicide Rates by Country

Suicides per 100,000 people

Rank		Country	Male	Female	Total	Year
1		Lithuania	70.1	14.0	40.2	2004
2		Belarus	63.3	10.3	35.1	2003
3		Russia	61.6	10.7	34.3	2004
4		Kazakhstan	51.0	8.9	29.2	2003
5		Hungary	44.9	12.0	27.7	2003
6		Guyana	42.5	12.1	27.2	2003
7		South Korea	N/A	N/A	26.1	2005
8		Slovenia	37.9	13.9	25.6	2004
9		Latvia	42.9	8.5	24.3	2004
10		Japan	35.6	12.8	24.0	2004

Source: The World Health Organization, 2005.

to the difference in lifestyles in this country can be overwhelming. There are conflicts that may arise due to language barriers or not speaking English, the dominant language. This stress encountered by the foreign-born has been related to depression and suicidal thoughts, especially among college students trying to fit in. In fact, young Latina girls not born in this country have high rates of suicide attempts, according to the Centers for Disease Control and Prevention (CDC).

Some immigrants may develop low self-esteem and feelings of isolation due to social alienation and marginalization. These are two conditions that can be correlated with suicidality or suicidal behavior. Social alienation refers to individuals feelings of not belonging or drifting apart from their community or peers. Often their relationships are shallow or superficial. Marginalization refers to being excluded from participation because it is believed that an individual could not participate to full capacity; for example, not being picked to play on a team because you are a girl. Groups such as individuals living with disabilities (physical or mental), girls, racial minorities, elderly individuals, teen mothers, and homosexuals may all face certain forms of marginalization.

SEXUAL ORIENTATION

Gays, lesbians, bisexuals, transgendered people, and people in question about their sexuality are at extreme risk for suicide. This population faces **stigma** (a negative mark against someone), discrimination, and are often victims of violence. It is difficult to determine if some of the suicides among young males are due to their sexual orientation because the family may not want to divulge that information or may not know at all. One mother who was very outspoken about her son's suicide had this to say:

> Joshua's suicide could have been because he was being teased at school about his sexuality. The kids made fun of his tight jeans and the way he wore his hair. He liked to wear long braids like the American Indians. Joshua was 15 when he took his own life, and we were never sure whether he was gay or not. I don't think he was certain himself, but the teasing at school frustrated him.

The CDC notes that young gay males are two to three times more likely than their peers to attempt suicide. Some evidence suggests lesbians have higher rates of smoking, being overweight, alcohol abuse, and stress than heterosexual women. The issues surrounding personal, family, and social acceptance of sexual orientation can place a significant burden on mental health and personal safety, which can be pathways to suicidal behavior.

TEENS SPEAK

I Knew I Was Gay

I knew I was gay from the very beginning. I just had a hard time living life, and once I decided to take my own. I was teased by my peers in elementary school and throughout high school. It just wouldn't stop. Middle school had to be the worst three years of my life. As soon as I walked in the room, people knew who I was. "Look! There goes the faggot! Faggot! Faggot! Faggot!" they would yell. And I grew insecure. I felt like everyone knew who I was because I got the feeling that all eyes were on me and the whispering voices were about me whether I walked in the classroom or in the cafeteria. I had a high-pitched voice in middle school, just like any other 11-year-old boy. That was the number one reason kids would tease me. I also didn't have that many friends. I tried to find excuses to sit out of gym class because I wasn't very athletic, that was reason number two. By the time I was in eighth grade, everyone knew who I was and knew me as the "queer one."

I was so relieved when high school started. I thought I would begin a new life, meet new people, and overcome painful memories. Unfortunately, half of the student body in my eighth grade class ended up going to the same high school I did. I thought things would be better, but it became worse once new faces whispered, "He's gay, he's gay." I knew right then and there that my old classmates gossiped to new friends about me. History would repeat itself. But thankfully, I made new friends and was one of the popular Hispanic students since I was captain of the Latin dance group. I came out to my peers the summer after sophomore year. I felt it was time for a new start, and thought it was funny how the ones who made fun of me began to be nice to me once I came out.

I started having suicidal thoughts after watching Kelly Rowland's music video *Stole.* [In this video, a young male takes his own life. The video shows how the other students reacted with great sorrow and regrets.] I thought to myself, "Would anyone care if I shot myself in the bathroom? Would people tell the reporters that I was never accepted because they treated me like dirt? How would they feel? Would they regret saying those nasty awful things to me?" Not just killing myself in school, I also thought about shooting my enemies and then killing myself, just like the school shootings that have happened in the past. One time, I had thoughts about turning to witchcraft so that my enemies can suffer as I have. But as I continued doing research, every spell would indicate, "Be careful, harming another would come back three times as bad." I definitely did not want to take that path. I was trapped: I didn't know what to do.

Now that I am in college, I feel so great about myself. Coming out to the world seemed like the right thing to do. Who cares what people think about you? You do! My friends helped me a lot. Friends are there for you because they love you and want to look out for you. They are there to help you, not to judge you. Taking your own life away will not solve anything; it'll make things worse. Do you want to see your mother crying every single day of her life because her child decided to be a coward and take his or her life? It's not going to help!

I've learned that you change your life by changing the way you think. You control your life. Don't let anyone put you down just because you are overweight, suffering from acne, homosexual, or the biggest nerd in school. One thing I've learned: move on with your life and live it day by day. Let karma take care of your enemies.

See also: Mental Illness and Suicide; Suicide and the Gay, Lesbian, Bisexual, and Transgender Communities

FURTHER READING

Joiner, Thomas. *Why People Die by Suicide.* Cambridge, Mass.: Harvard University Press, 2005.

■ CYBERSUICIDE
See: Internet Suicide

■ DRUGS AND SUICIDE
See: Alcohol, Drugs, and Suicide

■ DEPRESSION AND SUICIDE
See: Mental Illness and Suicide

■ ETHNICITY AND SUICIDE
Completed suicides, in which people take their own lives, and suicide attempts vary widely across different populations and across ethnic groups in the United States. Like completed suicides, suicide attempts are

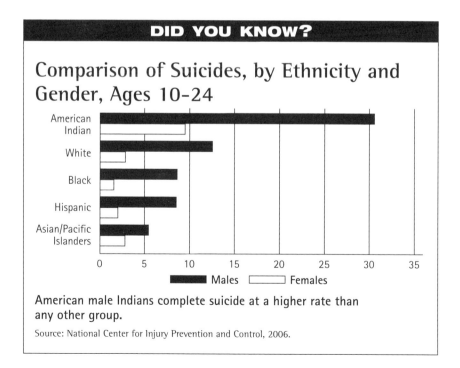

DID YOU KNOW?

Comparison of Suicides, by Ethnicity and Gender, Ages 10-24

American male Indians complete suicide at a higher rate than any other group.

Source: National Center for Injury Prevention and Control, 2006.

also self-inflicted destructive acts with the explicit intent to die, but they are nonfatal. Generally, whites and American Indians have the highest suicide rates. Suicide varies among diverse populations by method, location, intent, diagnoses, and demographics. For example, while African-American males have higher rates of suicide among young adults, white males have higher rates of suicide among men in middle age.

AMERICAN INDIANS

According to the National Adolescent Health Information Center, in 2005, the suicide rates for young American Indian males was two to four times that of young males in other racial and ethnic categories. Because there are more than 250 different languages spoken within the American Indian community, customs and attitudes toward mental health vary widely from one tribal group to another. This is true even for tribes within the same geographic region, such as in Oklahoma, which hosts 38 different tribes and the largest American Indian population in the United States.

AFRICAN AMERICANS

The rate of suicide among African Americans had historically been lower than that of whites; however, in the 1980s, the rate of suicide among young black males increased substantially. The suicide rates increased the most for blacks 10 to 14 years of age, at a rate of 233 percent. The trend reversed in the mid-1990s, and the suicide rate among young African-American males aged 15 to 24 years has steadily declined since 1994, but the rate has never been as low as it once was. African-American women have the lowest rate of suicide among all ethnic groups in the United States. In recent studies, it has been noted that black Americans have suicidal thoughts and behavior almost equal to that of the general population. However, generally speaking, African-American women are not reaching the level of hopelessness that leads to a completed suicide. There are no conclusive studies that explain why this is possible; speculative theories suggest that perhaps African-American women's socialization or life processes are more relational. In other words, they have closer family and community ties.

Q & A

Question: Why do black females have such low rates of suicide compared to everyone else?

Answer: Researchers are not totally certain, but they have speculated that African-American females have higher rates of resiliency. According to 2005 National Vital Statistics Reports, African-American females have the lowest suicide rate, while 5 percent of every 100,000 white females commit suicide. There also may be the religious factor among older black women. Studies have shown that black women have a tendency to refer their problems to God. Studies also indicate that African Americans in general come from larger families, have more responsibilities, and therefore feel less isolated and empty.

LATINOS

There has been little research on suicide in the Latino community. As a result, statistical data necessary to understand suicide among Latinos is limited. However, in the 2003 Youth Risk Behavioral Surveillance System, Latino students were more likely than white students to have reported a suicide attempt. Also, Latino students were more likely to have made a suicide plan than white males. Latino female students were significantly more likely than white female students to attempt suicide and require medical attention.

Researchers have found that among Latinos with mental **disorders**, fewer than one in 11 contact mental health specialists, while fewer than one in five contact general health-care providers. Among Latino immigrants with mental disorders, fewer than one in 20 use services from mental-health specialists, while fewer than one in 10 use services from general health-care providers.

ASIAN AMERICANS AND/OR PACIFIC ISLANDERS

Current data on suicide in Asian-American communities indicates rates of 5.5 percent for all age and ethnic subgroups. However, the data may be underreported, as it is calculated on the total Asian-American population, whereas suicide may be prevalent to a greater degree in particular ethnicities within the Asian-American category. For instance, suicide rates in a 20-year span (1970–90) rose 54 percent for Japanese American teenagers and 36 percent for Chinese American teenagers.

In 2000, suicide ranked as the second leading cause of death among Asian and Pacific Islander males ages 15 to 24 in the United States, according to the 2002 National Vital Statistics Report, the latest available data. According to the same report, Asian-American women ages 15 to 24 have a slightly higher rate of suicide than whites, blacks, and Hispanics in the same age group. Asian-American children and adolescents are considered by mental health providers to be highly prone to **depression.**

In a national survey, 30 percent of Asian-American girls in grades five to 12 reported suffering from depressive symptoms. Also, Asian-American girls reported the highest rates of depressive symptoms compared to white, black, and Hispanic girls. Asian-American teenage boys were more likely than their white, black, and Hispanic peers to report physical or sexual abuse. Asian-American children received less mental-health care than whites, blacks, and Hispanics.

See also: Culture and Suicide; Gender and Suicide

FURTHER READING

Bachman, Ronet. *Death and Violence on the Reservation: Homicide, Family Violence, and Suicide in American Indian Populations.* Westport, Conn.: Auburn House, 1992.

Lester, David. *Suicide in African Americans.* New York: NOVA Science, 1998.

———. *Suicide in American Indians.* New York: NOVA Science, 2001.

■ FAMILIES AND OTHER SURVIVORS

The effects of a suicide, the taking of one's own life, on parents, siblings, family members, and friends. Suicide is not a victimless crime. A suicide always leaves in its wake those loved ones left behind to suffer the loss, the guilt, and to wonder if they had anything to do with the decision to commit suicide. When someone commits suicide to get rid of internal pain, it is not over. The pain for the loved ones left behind just begins. Suicide survivors are those who have lost a family member or close friend to suicide. Losing a child to suicide is a parent's worst nightmare. The emotional turmoil that follows is extremely complex. Surviving family members may experience guilt, shame, blame, and anger. You can never really know why someone has died by suicide, even when he or she leaves a note. But one can speculate. Ten to 15 percent of suicides leaves notes—a small percentage. The notes are often short and cryptic, which still leaves families wondering why.

Most families and friends are not content until they get to the bottom of why their loved one suicided. They will search the literature, read all the books, talk with others who have experienced the same type of death in their family, and look for support. Some go to therapy and get counseling on how to get through the grieving process. Each day they face the painful struggle of asking themselves why. If you lose someone in a car accident, you have answers, just as you do if you lose someone to a **terminal illness.** After a suicide, the person is dead and you cannot ask them anything. As mentioned, notes left behind are often unclear. To help get through the pain of suicide, many families need to talk about it. Often, survivors experience a feeling of greater grief around the dates of the suicide—a condition known as an **anniversary reaction.** Survivors may also be struck with **delayed grief,** bereavement that occurs years or decades after the loss.

Q & A

Question: Will talking about suicide make someone take his or her own life?

Answer: No, talking to a person about suicide will not make that person try it. Talking about suicide lets a person know he or she is not alone and that you care. Most people are relieved to finally be able to talk about their feelings, and this alone will reduce the risk of an attempt. *Not* talking about suicide makes it impossible to prevent. You cannot prevent what you do not know.

SUPPORT GROUPS

There are hundreds of support groups all over the country, primarily designed for those who have lost a loved one to suicide. One support group in Washington, D.C., limits membership to families who have lost someone to suicide. People who lose someone to suicide have a different pain that goes beyond normal grief. In a panel discussion at a national conference, one 21-year-old woman explained how her mother had jumped from the roof of a hospital in New York City. What she could not understand is why her mother had decided to put her daughter's shoes on before she jumped. "She was wearing my shoes!" exclaimed the young woman as she broke into tears.

Another woman who lost her 15-year-old son to suicide explains how she heard a thump coming from her son's bedroom at 4:00 in the morning and went back to sleep. Around 7:30 A.M., she decided to go to his room to get him up for school and found him dead on the floor after hanging himself. She is racked with guilt that she did not check on him when she heard the thump. She feels she may have been able to revive him and save him.

There are families who attend support groups because they find it more comforting than one-on-one therapy. They want to talk about the suicide, and a therapist may instead want them to talk about how they are getting through the grieving process—whether they are sleeping okay and eating well. Survivors of a suicide need to get through their anger and **denial** by talking about the suicide—especially with those who have experienced it. One woman whose 20-year-old son drove his car into a river did not want to talk to anyone unless they lost a 20-year-old son to suicide. Survivors need to know they are not alone.

A SafePlace in Boston, Massachusetts, is a support group founded in 1971. There were families in that area that lost loved ones to suicide, and they had no place to go where others would understand their grief. SafePlace has no agenda, no speakers, no required readings, and although people may look for them, no answers, explains George Howe Colt in *The Enigma of Suicide,* published in 1992. There is just a lot of talk, talk, and more talk from each attendee. It is generally open for any discussion. The goal, Colt explains, is to create an atmosphere in which people can safely grieve with no one passing judgment. Many survivors suffer from ongoing **chronic grief.** The condition of experiencing an abnormal grief reaction after the loss of deeply dependent relationship is known as **chronic grief syndrome.**

GETTING THROUGH THE GUILT

A person should not feel guilty about what he or she did not know. The woman who heard the thump coming from her son's bedroom did not know that he had just hanged himself. She had no idea, which is why she rolled over and went back to sleep.

The term *acute suicide threat* is used to describe someone who has the lethal means to end his or her own life and has threatened to do so. Even if you know they may kill themselves, you are not a superhero and cannot save everybody. At a survival support group, one mother explained how her son had been in the kitchen trying to stab himself with a knife. She grabbed the knife from him, and he ran out the back door, jumped over the fence; she ran through another yard. The mother tried to run after him but could not jump over the fence, she ran up the street and around the block until she could find him. She turned a corner and found him hanging from a lamppost. Did she feel guilty? Yes, she did. Could she have saved him? Does not seem like it. There are times when individuals really want to die, and they will, either through killing themselves or getting killed by another. According to the American Association of Suicidology, some researchers found that about 10 percent or more of the total suicides cannot be saved because they take their lives in such a way that it was impossible to have saved them.

Q & A

Question: Is it more likely for a person to attempt suicide if they have been exposed to it in their family?

Answer: We know that suicide can run in families, but studies have indicated that this is due to the fact that **depression** and related depressive illnesses have a genetic or hereditary component. It is the mental disorder that can be passed on, *not* the actual act of a suicide. Talking about suicide or being aware of a suicide that happened in your family does not put you at risk for attempting it, especially if you are mentally healthy. The only family members at risk are those who are vulnerable in the first place—vulnerable because of an illness of depression or another depressive illnesses. The risk increases if the illness is not treated. It is important to remember that not all people who have depression have suicidal thoughts—only some.

DENIAL

The woman whose 20-year-old son drove his car into the river had two children before his death, and now she has one. For months she could not bring herself to refer to only one child and kept referring to "the kids." "I have to get home and fix dinner for the kids," she would say. She would not allow anyone to go into her son's room and remove anything. He had left change on his nightstand—a couple of dimes and a quarter. It stayed there. When her daughter needed some change, she started to go to his room and get a dime, and the mother told her not to touch the change in his room (as though he would be back one day). Others try to erase all traces of the dead person from the house, getting rid of all their possessions, never mentioning his or her name again, as in the case of Stanley Kunitz, taken from the *Enigma of Suicide* in his poem "The Portrait":

> *My Mother never forgave my father for killing himself, . . . When I came down from the attic with the pastel portrait in my hand of a long-lipped stranger with a brave moustache and deep brown level eyes, she ripped it into shreds without a single word. . . .*

A well-known actress explains that her son did not kill himself . . . it was an accident. She explained how he had called her on the phone, was very distraught about something, and had a gun in his hand. He told her he was cleaning it. Then she heard it go off, and he was dead. She insists he shot himself accidentally. Perhaps it was an accident, perhaps she is in denial.

MISTAKEN ASSUMPTIONS

The American Association of Suicidology explains in their handbook for survivors of suicide that suicide survivors are prone to many negative assumptions that are likely to be false, such as:

- "I know why they did it." The motivations behind suicide are multifaceted or complex. It is never one reason but usually a number of things.

- "If I'd only done such and such, they'd still be alive." Thinking that you or anyone else could have prevented the suicide is assuming that we all have far more power over the lives of others than we actually do. Furthermore, many suicide victims persist and persist until they succeed.

- "It's their girlfriend's fault; or their boyfriend's fault; or their parents' fault." Blaming others is a form of denial. Only by facing the truth of your loss and the responsibility that lies with the victim can you recover from grief.

- "I will never be able to enjoy life again." Don't deny your mind's natural ability to heal. While your life may be forever changed, it need not be forever painful.

LOSING A FRIEND TO SUICIDE

Losing a friend, a boyfriend, or a girlfriend to suicide is detrimental, especially at a young age. Some wonder why a suicide victim did not tell anyone that he or she wanted to die or that the victim did not express his or her pain to anyone, and those in wonderment feel betrayed. Some people feel guilty because they did not notice the signs of a friend's suicidal thoughts. A college student explains that he should have known his friend was going to kill herself when she gave him her book bag in the middle of the semester. Some get very angry at others who were closer to the victim for not being there for them. Some are racked with guilt. Most parents who lose a child to suicide want their child's friends to be around them because it brings them closer to their dead child. The friends become extensions of the deceased.

If you have lost a friend to suicide, it may help to stay in touch with the family; it may help you and the family. However, if the family is blaming you, seek help to discuss the situation with a professional. Do not internalize the blame to the point where you believe the accusations. Be open to discussion with others who knew the victim until the family begins to heal. Blaming yourself is part of the healing process when a loved one takes his or her own life. Some survivors feel the need to point the finger at someone because it helps them with the "why." It gives them a false sense of relief if they can say it is someone's fault.

WHAT'S MENTIONABLE IS MANAGEABLE

Suicide need not be crippling if it is discussed openly and honestly. The more family and friends gather to talk about their loved one who completed suicide–the better. Not talking about it means that the pain is being internalized. Once pain is internalized, it can manifest in other ways and when least expected, oftentimes through emotional outburst, unexplained anger, or withdrawal. Talking it out helps; support groups help. Talking about the loved one could mean remembering the good things, remembering how much he or she made you laugh, remembering his or her smile, quirks, and funny expressions. It does not always have to be about the pain–though it is important to get through the pain.

See also: Culture and Suicide; Gender and Suicide

FURTHER READING

Bolton, Iris. *My Son . . . My Son: A Guide to Healing After Death, Loss, or Suicide.* Rev. ed. Roswell, Ga.: Bolton Press Atlanta, 1983.

Cammarta, Doreen. *Someone I Loved Died by Suicide: A Story for Child Survivors and Those Who Care for Them.* Palm Beach Gardens, Fla.: Florida Grief Guidance, 2001.

Cobain, Beverly, and Jean Larch. *Dying to Be Free: A Healing Guide for Families After a Suicide.* Center City, Minn.: Hazelden, 2006.

Fine, Carla. *No Time to Say Goodbye.* New York: Broadway Books, 1997.

Reynolds, Michael. *Surviving Bill.* Lincoln, Nebr.: iUniverse Books, 2007.

■ GENDER AND SUICIDE

The biological differences between males and females and the effect of those differences on suicide, or the taking of one's own life, and suicide attempts. While boys complete suicide more than girls, girls

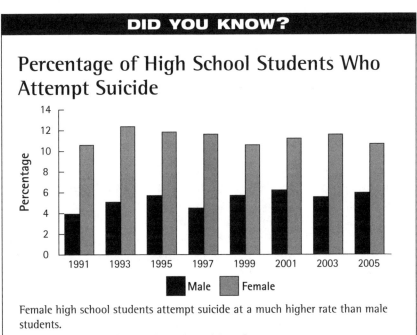

DID YOU KNOW?

Percentage of High School Students Who Attempt Suicide

Female high school students attempt suicide at a much higher rate than male students.

Source: National Center for Injury Prevention and Control, 2006.

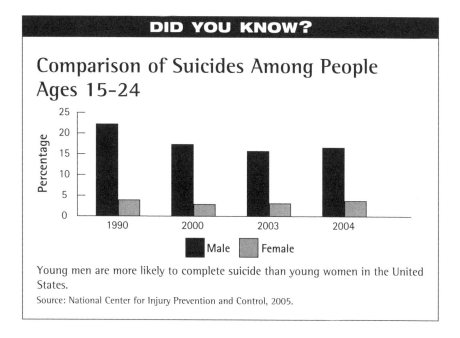

DID YOU KNOW?

Comparison of Suicides Among People Ages 15-24

Young men are more likely to complete suicide than young women in the United States.

Source: National Center for Injury Prevention and Control, 2005.

attempt suicide more than boys. Some of the underlying reasons for such a large gap between sexes revolve around the risk factors. Risk factors are those factors that put someone at risk for suicide or those lifestyles that put someone in danger for completing suicide. Alcohol abuse and substance abuse can put someone at risk for suicide. Access to firearms can put someone at risk for suicide.

Young boys have a higher risk for suicide because they engage in alcohol abuse more than young girls do. Also, according to national surveillances conducted by the Centers for Disease Control (CDC), boys have more access to guns than girls. If boys suffer from **depression,** they will not seek help as quickly as girls do. Oftentimes, a suicide is completed because of impulsive tendencies and aggressive tendencies. Boys have higher rates of aggressive and impulsive behavior. Girls are more likely to engage in suicidal behavior using **medications** that could cause an overdose. Furthermore, girls are less likely to use alcohol during a suicide attempt. Alcohol could lead to more violent means, such as increasing the chances for use of a gun to complete a suicide.

Also, the reasoning for suicide can differ between boys and girls. For instance, boys are much more likely than girls to have experienced a crisis in the 24-hour period before their death. This includes things such as being arrested for the first time, having to appear in court, or being publicly humiliated.

GENDER SOCIALIZATION

Girls are reared differently from boys. Their toys are different, the colors they are associated with at birth are different, and parents often treat boys and girls differently. Boys' toys and games are more competitive—there is generally a winner and a loser with their toys from racecars to sports. Hence, the aggressive behavior to win! Girls' toys such as dolls are passive, quiet, and gentle. Because girls are socialized differently than boys, the behavior between the two sexes varies. The lifelong social experience by which males and females develop their human potential plays a major factor in how they act or react to certain situations

Silvia Canetto, author of *Love and Achievement Motives in Women's and Men's Suicide Notes,* argues that females, as a result of how they are reared or socialized, may have different ways of coping, and males, because of how they are reared, see things in a more aggressive manner and like to do things with a winning result such as suicide. The thought is, "If I am going to take my own life—I am going to do it in a way that will make it a sure thing." It is a macho attitude that places an emphasis on not failing. Females who were raised to be nurturing have less of a problem with seeking help from other females. It is not viewed as a sign of weakness because talking about your problems with others is considered to be a female trait. Men and boys view help-seeking behavior as "girly," or a sign of weakness. Boys are told not to cry, not to show their feelings, and told not to be a "wuss." They are raised to believe that they should be able to handle their problems on their own and provide their own solutions.

Dr. William Pollack, author of *Real Boys,* writes: "Research shows that male infants are more emotionally expressive than female infants. However, as a boy ages, his emotional expressiveness decreases. Why? Because of society's definition of what it means to be a boy. Society demands that boys cover up their emotions. And as a result, boys develop a 'mask of masculinity' to hide their shame, vulnerability, and the other feelings they cannot express publicly. The inability to show true emotions hardens a boy until he loses touch with them."

As these boys grow older, they show no fear of violence, adhere to being macho, and believe teasing others is acceptable behavior. The emotion they *can* express that will keep them being macho is anger. All this can contribute to more violent behavior in boys, such as getting into fights, drinking and drugging, and taking their own lives. This is believed to be the reason for such higher rates of suicide among boys.

GENDER DIFFERENCES IN OTHER COUNTRIES

According to the World Health Organization (WHO), in western nations such as Greece, Mexico, and the United States, male suicides outnumber the female suicides. However, in some Asian nations there tends to be less of a gap. There are even parts of China where the rate of female suicides is higher than males.

Every year in China, 1.5 million women attempt to take their own lives, and 150,000 complete suicide. Suicide is three times higher in the rural areas than in the cities. One reason given is that poisons and pesticides are readily available in the agricultural regions. As women routinely choose less violent means of suicide, the presence of these deadly chemicals increases the risk factor for women committing suicide.

Also, many marriages in rural areas are still arranged and occur at a very early age. The groom's parents "buy the bride," in which the parents of the bride from rural poor areas sell her, and she becomes part of their family. This leads to emotional problems for

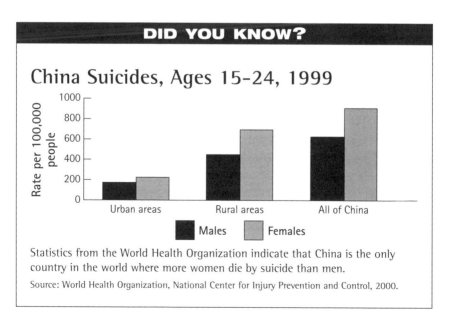

DID YOU KNOW?

China Suicides, Ages 15–24, 1999

Statistics from the World Health Organization indicate that China is the only country in the world where more women die by suicide than men.

Source: World Health Organization, National Center for Injury Prevention and Control, 2000.

young wives who are forced into an alien environment. Arguments and violence often occur in arranged marriages where the young woman is not happy about the arrangement and rendered powerless. Leaving the marriage is generally not an option for the woman because she will have disgraced her family and will be ostracized. Xu Rong, head of the Suicide Prevention Project at the Beijing Cultural Development Centre for Rural Women, estimates that 70 to 80 percent of suicides are the direct result of conflicts between husbands and wives. Further studies have indicated that there are low rates of depression among those who died by suicide, and other studies have shown that the suicide trend among young women results from the experience of interpersonal and financial crises and not so much from a mental illness.

According to a national study conducted by the CDC, among 895 suicide victims, researchers found that only 63 percent of the victims suffered from a mental illness. The most common negative life event in the year before their death was financial problems, a serious physical illness, and marital conflict. The suicides tended to be impulsive acts of drinking poison or pesticides. A study at Central University of Finance and Economics in Beijing, China, found that gender inequality was largely a reason that women attempted and completed suicide. Greater value is placed on boys than girls. In China, the frame of mind that compels someone to take his or her own life differs from that of the United States. In this country, suicide is caused more as result of hopelessness and depression. In China, there is a traditional belief that suicide is honorable for those in a desperate situation and are powerless to escape. You do not have to be mentally ill to kill yourself. The society in China offers suicide as an "acceptable" option, according to Michael Phillips, who has been studying the high rates of suicide in China.

However, there are other countries in which the male rate of suicide is much higher than that of females, such as in the United States, where males kill themselves at a rate of four times that of females. In other countries such as Belarus the rate of male suicides to females can be five or six times higher. According to the 2008 WHO data, Lithuania had 68 male and 13 female suicides per 100,000 people. Belarus had the second-highest rate, with 63 males and 10 females per 100,000 people.

See also: Ethnicity and Suicide; Suicide and the Gay, Lesbian, Bisexual, and Transgender Communities

FURTHER READING

Canetto, Silvia. "Love and Achievement Motives in Women's and Men's Suicide Notes." *Journal of Psychology* 136, no. 5 (2002).

Leach, Mark. *Cultural Diversity and Suicide: Ethnic, Religious, Gender and Sexual Orientation Perspectives.* New York: Routledge, 2006.

■ GRIEF AND MOURNING

See: Families and Other Survivors

■ GUILT AND SUICIDE

See: Families and Other Survivors

■ HOMICIDE AND SUICIDE

A situation in which someone kills another and then himself or herself, also known as **murder-suicide.** There are several theories as to why murder-suicide occurs. Sometimes the perpetrator is facilitating a mass murder, as in suicide bombings. The person may also be trying to escape punishment or inflict self-punishment due to guilt. There are also cases in which the assailants set out to kill themselves but planned on a murder first; for example: murdering their children first or a family member first; committing joint suicide with someone who has consented; or taking revenge out on those who hurt them, such as an ex-girlfriend or boyfriend or bullies at school.

The motivation for the murder in a murder-suicide can be purely suicidal in many cases. In other words, many times the ultimate goal of a murder-suicide is suicide itself. A suicide can follow a murder sometimes out of guilt, but many times it occurs because of hopelessness to the point where life no longer has any meaning, and the killer wants also to kill those whom he or she feels contributed to a seemingly meaningless life. In many murder-suicide cases, an individual could be suffering from aggressive rage that is internalized (taking it out on self, therefore, a suicide) or rage that is externalized (taking it out on others, therefore, a homicide).

Studies have shown that many murder-suicides are committed by persons with borderline personality, psychotic, or schizophrenic traits.

More than 50 percent of persons studied have alcohol in their system. A suicidal college student took the lives of 32 people at Virginia Tech before turning the gun on himself in 2007. The following year, another suicidal student took the lives of five others before killing himself at Northern Illinois University. In 1999, there was a high school shooting at Columbine High School in Colorado at which 12 students and one teacher were killed and 23 others wounded in the nation's deadliest school shooting. Two suicidal students had plotted for a year to kill at least 500 people and blow up their school. At the end of their hour-long rampage, they turned their guns on themselves. This is a classic example of taking revenge on those deemed responsible for the pain and suffering the shooters were going through and then escaping the world, which is seen as a terrible place.

There are also people who kill family members first and then take their own lives. Where suicide is generally the main act, oftentimes murdering one's own children or spouse first takes place. It is believed that in cases like this the suicidal person wants to keep his or her children from being without a parent and spare the family from a horrible life in general. The person feels that life has no meaning and therefore will have no meaning for the children. There are also cases in which it is never known why an individual would want to kill his or her family before killing him or herself—as in the case of the well-known Canadian professional wrestler Christopher Michael Benoit.

Benoit wrestled for Extreme Championship Wrestling (ECW), World Championship Wrestling (WCW), and World Wrestling Entertainment (WWE). He rose to the top of his profession, holding the World Heavyweight Championship in both WCW and WWE, becoming one of the most popular and respected competitors in professional wrestling in the process. Chris, his wife, Nancy, and their seven-year-old son, Daniel, were found dead in their home in Fayetteville, Georgia, on June 25, 2007. Authorities confirmed that Benoit killed his wife and son and subsequently hanged himself. After the double murder-suicide, former wrestler Chris Nowinski contacted Michael Benoit, father of Chris Benoit, suggesting that years of trauma to his son's brain may have led to his actions. Tests were conducted on Benoit's brain by Julian Bailes, the head of neurosurgery at West Virginia University, and results showed that "Benoit's brain was so severely damaged it resembled the brain of an 85-year-old Alzheimer's patient." He was also shown to have an advanced form of dementia, and his brain was similar to the brains of four retired NFL players who had suffered multiple concussions, sank into **depression,** and harmed themselves or others. Bailes and his colleagues concluded that repeated concussions can lead to dementia, which can contribute to severe behavioral problems. Benoit's father suggested that brain damage may have been the leading cause of his crime.

WHAT HAPPENED AT RED LAKE?

A young teen on the Red Lake Reservation in Minnesota went on a shooting rampage in March 2005. He killed his grandparents first, traveled to the Red Lake school, killing nine people, then turned the gun on himself. According to a Minnesota Public Radio special report entitled *What Happens at Red Lake,* members of the Indian tribe on the Red Lake Reservation in northern Minnesota strive to protect their Ojibwe culture, traditions, and language. The Red Lake Reservation is as large as it was in the 19th century. Red Lake never traded away its land, and parcels of land cannot be sold to outsiders. This allows for the tribe to hold on to traditions and pass them on. They still practice the same ceremonies their ancestors practiced long before Europeans arrived in North America. These ceremonies cannot be easily understood by outsiders because they are not a fixed event that can easily be explained, but a living, breathing extension of the people who are participating.

Unfortunately, only about half of the enrolled members of the tribe at Red Lake Reservation live on the reservation at one time. In fact, many families live part of their life in the Twin Cities—Minneapolis or St. Paul. Jeff Weise, the teen shooter, lived most of the time in the city, away from the reservation, where there were traditional practices, spiritual beliefs, and cultural survival. What the city residents search for is a connection to a community.

It is essential for these young American Indians to have their identity, know where they come from, and be able to practice their traditional culture. The Red Lake School is nearly 100 percent Indian with only 1 percent of the teaching staff being of the heritage. Truancy was high and attendance low, therefore grades were also low. Some feel that the children were disrespected, ignored, and forgotten. In general, children do not attend or go to a place where they are not comfortable. Under the guidance of elders, traditional healers, teachers, and counselors, Red Lake is trying to begin a process so that the children will not become disconnected from their roots as Weise did. His murder-suicide was caused by feelings of alienation and rage at his situation. This rage was transferred to others and then to himself.

SUICIDE PACTS

A suicide pact describes the suicides of two or more individuals in an agreed-upon plan. The plan may be to die together, or separately and closely timed. Suicide pacts are important concepts to researchers and health-care experts who study suicide, as they have occurred throughout history, as well as in fiction.

Suicide pacts are generally distinct from **mass suicides.** The latter refers to incidents in which a larger number of people kill themselves together for the same ideological reason, often within a religious, political, military, or paramilitary context. Suicide pacts, on the other hand, usually involve small groups of people (such as married or romantic partners, family members, or friends) whose motivations are intensely personal and individual. A suicide pact negotiated over the Internet, often between complete strangers, is an Internet suicide.

A classic example of a suicide pact occurred in New England in 1994, when a husband and wife agreed that the husband would shoot the wife, who was dying of cancer, and then the husband, who was getting old and feeble, would shoot himself. The man succeeded in killing his wife but shot himself and wound up hospitalized. When he woke up and found out he had botched the job, he was very upset. His children were even more upset that their parents had made the pact. Eventually, the father went to live with one of his children.

WARNING SIGNS

It is difficult to determine when individuals are going to go into a homicidal rage and take the lives of those around them. Again, most of the cases of people on school grounds or universities also took their own life. It is believed these were suicidal students. They wanted to kill themselves but not before taking others out with them. The warning signs do not differ from the general warning signs of a suicidal person. Warning signs are those signals that individuals will give when they are in a suicidal or homicidal crisis. A suicidal crisis occurs when a person is thinking and planning to take his or her own life or actually getting ready to attempt suicide, whereas a homicidal crisis is just the opposite. The person in crisis is thinking and planning to take someone else's life as well as his or her own perhaps but not always. At this point, a person begins giving out all sorts of signs. Signals vary, and there is rarely just one signal, but several. Three main warning signs that need to be taken seriously include:

- someone threatening to hurt someone, or talking of wanting to hurt someone
- someone looking for ways to hurt another person, such as obtaining access to firearms or other means
- someone talking or writing about death and homicide, when these actions are out of the ordinary for the person

When a student withdraws, is isolated, constantly being picked on by others, and is considered being different from others, he or she has to be suffering from pain. It is painful not to be included, to be considered a "weirdo," to be picked on by others through name calling, being pushed or shoved, and being talked about. The warnings signs are not found so much in how such people act as much as how they are being treated by others. The pain is internalized and can be manifested through frustration, anger, aggressive and violent behavior, substance abuse, and impulsiveness.

See also: Ethnicity and Suicide; Families and Other Survivors

■ INTERNET SUICIDE (CYBERSUICIDE)

A visibly interactive taking of one's life, a suicide in which an individual involves others on the World Wide Web to view the event. The Internet is a phenomenon with little to no boundaries. Taking one's own life in a public display is currently rare. A suicide of this nature leaves little room for intervention and serves as a form of perverted entertainment for those watching on their computers. The public show, in which the individual putting on the display writes the script and does the performing, can be a form of mockery, not taking the suicide or the internal pain that one is suffering seriously.

In a 2008 case involving a 19-year-old male, viewers watched for several hours as the victim appeared to be sleeping after ingesting a number of pills. One viewer finally called the authorities, who then contacted the moderator of the site to obtain the location of the victim. By the time the authorities reached the location, it was too late. Laws and policies are currently being formulated so that using this method of suicide can be prevented in the future.

There is also what is known as an Internet suicide pact, in which individuals who meet over the Internet decide together to take their own lives. The first known Internet suicide pact took place in Japan in October 2000. Cases following were said to be reported in China, South Korea, Australia, Sweden, and the United States. According to the May 2005 issue of the *Christchurch School of Medicine,* in New Zealand, an article entitled "Canterbury Suicide Project" found that a growing number of Internet suicide pacts involve young people who are generally complete strangers or individuals with simple friendships with the common characteristic between them being clinical depression.

See also: Cluster Suicides; Homicide and Suicide

■ MANIC DEPRESSIVE DISORDER
See: Mental Illness and Suicide

■ MEDIA COVERAGE
The television, newspaper, Web, and radio news reports on suicide. Media reports on suicide can sometimes be too sensational, causing excitement, especially for those people already drawn toward suicidal behavior. It is not necessary for the media to cause such excitement by reporting a suicide in detail with graphics or startling impressions that please the gory, negative taste of individuals. Evidence suggests that an article or public story of a suicide, especially a celebrity, increases the number of completed and attempted suicides. This effect is called a contagion—a series of consecutive suicides influenced by either the media or a suicide by a well-known, influential individual. Because of this effect, experts in the field of suicide are making efforts to assist news reporters in the way they handle their stories. It is not necessarily the coverage of the suicide that causes contagion, but the way it is reported. If experts can change attitudes and reporting techniques within the media, there would likely be fewer cases of such deaths.

Interest in suicidal behavior tends to increase when the media report on cases of **assisted suicide,** in which a **terminally ill** patient is helped to commit suicide by a doctor or other medical professional. Assisted suicide is illegal in the United States, except in the states of Oregon and Washington. Under the Oregon Death with Dignity Act, patients of sound mind can request a prescription for a lethal dose of **medication.** Two doctors must confirm a diagnosis of terminal illness with no more than six months to live. Two witnesses, one of whom may be the original doctor and one nondoctor unrelated to the patient, or three total individuals, must confirm the patient's request. The patient must then make a second request after 15 days. The 2008 Washington law is closely modeled on the Oregon law, which was passed in 1994.

CHANGING THE COVERAGE OF SUICIDE

If a suicide is reported in the media, the reporter should not make it appear that the suicide can be explained simplistically. Often, the public wants to know why. Why did this person kill himself? What drove him to it? Reporters try to answer this question by focusing on one main event. However, suicide is never the result of a single event. There are a number of **stressors,** sometimes coupled with psychological or social problems or a mental **disorder.** It is best to let the public know that "Johnny didn't kill himself because he was suspended from school," but because Johnny had some other underlying problems that the public was not aware of and which compounded his stress. If the media focuses on one stressor as though that was what caused Johnny to suicide, then those in prevention and intervention will be looking for only one thing when trying to help a child who is suicidal. And once that one thing is taken care of, they think the problem is over.

Reporting the suicide over and over in the news causes a preoccupation with suicide among persons at risk or who are already vulnerable to suicide. These people have been thinking about it, contemplating it, and possibly making plans to suicide. Watching news coverage over and over about a suicide can open up old wounds and cause people to begin thinking about it more seriously. To decrease the chances that they are encouraging suicide among such people, reporters and news representatives need to review alternative ways to cover a newsworthy suicide story. The National Council for Suicide Prevention and the American Foundation for Suicide Prevention, as well as other organizations, insist that it is imperative to end a report on a celebrated suicide story with how to seek help and to list the number of the national suicide hotline in the top left corner of the screen on every frame during the report.

To further limit the contagion of suicide, news outlets have to omit sensationalism. The report should not be graphic, giving too much detail on the specifics of the suicide so as to draw attention to the manner of death; the story should not give chilling impressions.

As with repetition of the story, sensational reporting can also cause those previously preoccupied by suicide to begin thinking about it again. News reports should avoid photographs of the funeral, the dead body, the room in which the person slept, and so on. Too much attention to the act of suicide may make a person who is thinking of suicide go ahead with the idea in an effort to get attention—even though it will be after death.

When the glamorous actress of the 1950s Marilyn Monroe allegedly killed herself in 1962, there was constant reporting. The news showed the emergency medical team taking her body out of the house and the bed in which she was found dead. Shortly after, in the same month of her death, 197 more suicides were reported than would have been expected under normal circumstances.

Another danger is reporting on the method of suicide in detail. While viewers may want to know all the gory details, such reporting only puts ideas in the heads of the vulnerable people watching the report. Reporting that someone shot himself or herself is not necessarily harmful. However, stating in detail how the victim got hold of the gun, what position the gun was in when the shot was made, and where the bullets entered and exited the body is unnecessary. Actual procedures used by the victim may facilitate imitations of the suicidal behavior or copycat suicides.

Reporting on memorial services
Beyond the details of the suicide itself, the media also make a difference when it comes to covering funerals and public services. Reporting on public memorials or participating in such an event may cause additional suicides because it appears that the community is honoring the suicidal behavior of the deceased person and not just the person. Parents will often engage in this sort of public display to memorialize their loved one.

In Texas, a parent came to her dead son's school and gave away his clothes to his friends. Her son was one of the first of a cluster of suicides to die. The individuals who followed with their own suicides either knew of her son or were his friends. One student who died by suicide used a belt given to him by the mother of the first student. Parents of the following suicides were slightly upset that the parent of the first suicide drew so much attention to her son's suicide.

A mother in Massachusetts was distraught because the school would not allow her daughter's friends to place a plaque on a large tree at her school. She felt it was a fitting tribute to her lost child. However, the school did not want any vulnerable students who were contemplating suicide to think that they would be memorialized too and think that it was "pretty cool." The school had to take precautionary measures not to draw too much attention to the suicide.

Fact Or Fiction?

Only real stories of suicide in the media have an effect on the young population.

The Facts: Studies have shown an increase in suicide among young adults after a suicide is depicted in a soap opera or in a TV movie. Novels are included. David Phillips, a sociologist, coined the term *Werther Effect* to mean a potential increase in suicides following the suicide of a well-known character—fictitious or real. This term came from the novel *The Sorrows of Young Werther,* written by the German author Goethe more than 200 years ago, in which the fictional hero, Werther, takes his own life by putting a pistol to his head after a failed love affair. This novel had an effect on young European romantics who read the novel back in the late 1700s. Many of them dressed like Werther, adopted his romantic persona, and died like him, by a gunshot to the head. Because of this, the book was banned in many European countries.

ROMANTICIZING SUICIDE

Some elements in the reporting of suicides or in the storytelling can affect the impact. For instance, in the story line of *The Sorrows of Young Werther,* suicide was depicted in a romantic light. Researchers have found that the more a suicide is romanticized, the greater the chances of the story having a contagious effect, meaning that the story can cause suicides by those who have been thinking about it. However, when a suicide story line is characterized as a criminal act or due to a psychiatric disorder, there is no significant imitation of suicides or contagion effect.

According to the Suicide Prevention Resource Center, there are special situations that need more careful handling than others. Celebrity deaths by suicide are more likely than noncelebrity deaths to produce imitation. Although suicides by celebrities will receive a lot of coverage, it is important for the report not to let the glamour of the individual overshadow any mental health problems or use of **drugs**. The public needs to understand the connection, if any, to keep the death from being romanticized.

In covering **murder-suicides**, it is necessary to understand that the homicide often masks the suicide. Usually the person is in a suicidal state first and then decides to kill someone else before taking his or her own life. Feelings of **depression** and hopelessness are generally present beforehand.

It is also important that reporting on suicide pacts be accurate. They are not simply and explicitly the act of loving individuals who do not wish to be separated. Most often, these pacts involve an individual who is coercive and another who is extremely dependent. The one in control generally has power over the dependent individual and is extremely influential and can convince this person that life is not worth living. Pacts are no different than group suicides such as the one in Jonestown. There, cult leader Jim Jones convinced his followers that suicide was the only way to escape life on Earth and live in the hereafter. The followers believed their leader and took cyanide, just as an individual can believe the person who has power over him or her.

How the media help can prevent suicide
The media should report a suicide responsibly, so there is no sensationalizing, glorifying, or romanticizing the suicide. The media has a responsibility to provide the public with information, but there are ways to minimize the effect the report may have on vulnerable individuals. Beyond the impact a report may have on such individuals, there is an ethical obligation to the friends and families of the deceased to minimize the emotional pain caused by the media attention. Once a report of a suicide is given, news outlets can follow the report with a full disclosure on suicide prevention. They can provide basic information on how to prevent a suicide and how to intervene when someone is in a suicidal crisis. They can also provide a list of suicide hotlines throughout the country or one national suicide prevention hotline. The public can be given

the signs that point to an individual in trouble. Additional stories to watch are:

- trends in suicide rates
- recent treatment advances
- individual accounts of how treatment was life-saving
- accounts of people who overcame despair without attempting suicide
- myths about suicide
- warning signs of suicide
- actions that individuals can take to prevent suicide by others.

See also: Cults and Suicide; Warning Signs

FURTHER READING
Cobain, Beverly, and Jean Larch. *Dying to Be Free: A Healing Guide for Families After a Suicide.* Center City, Minn.: Hazelden, 2006.

■ MENTAL ILLNESS AND SUICIDE

Psychological disorders that cause distressful effects, which may include suicide attempts and suicide completions. Examples include severe **depression, bipolar disorder** (mainly mixed states or rapid cycling of mood swings), and **schizophrenia.**

DID YOU KNOW?

Teens and Depression

About 2.1 million teens, aged 12–17, experience a major depressive episode in a 12-month period.

For almost half of the teens, depression drastically reduced their abilities to deal with aspects of their daily lives.

Source: Substance Abuse and Mental Health Services Administration, 2006.

A major depressive illness is defined as being in an intensely unhappy and hopeless mood for a period of two weeks or longer or having loss of interest or pleasure for two weeks or longer coupled with four other symptoms; disturbed sleeping patterns, problems with energy, poor concentration, and poor self-image. In other words, if there has been a change in functioning, such as sleeping too much or too little, having no energy or too much energy, being unable to concentrate, eating too much or too little, or a change in other similar regular habits—along with a depressed mood that has lasted for two or more weeks—then these are warning signs of a mental **disorder.**

DEPRESSION AND SUICIDE

During the 1950s and 1960s, it was believed that children and adolescents did not experience depression. This belief was based on the work of psychiatrist Sigmund Freud, who defined depression as anger turned inward by what is known as the superego, and supposedly children and adolescents did not have a fully developed superego; therefore, they could not get clinically depressed. If children and adolescents were moody and sad, it was attributed to the pains of growing up. Suicides by children and teenagers were classified as pure accidents, and suicides were thought to be rare. However, today some depression among teens is almost as common as a cold. The National Institute of Mental Health estimates that one in five children suffer from depression, and the literature states that depression peaks in adolescence. In other words, if an individual has a predisposition to depression, it can manifest in their early to late teens.

It is not unusual for most teens to feel briefly depressed about situations or events—a failed relationship, a poor grade, or losing a football game—but the feeling passes as one regains a more positive frame of mind. However, the illness called "depression" generally last about two weeks or more and can become major depression or clinical depression. When a depressed state becomes major or clinical, it is described as a mood disorder by the medical community. It is a physical illness due to a chemical imbalance of the brain. It impairs an individual's overall emotional, physical, and behavioral abilities as well as cognitive abilities or how he or she sees the world and understands it.

Most adolescent sadness is caused by a reaction to an event such as the poor grade rather than a chemical imbalance. These periods of sadness are brief and come at a time of going through an adolescent identity crisis–trying to figure out how to get from childhood to adulthood–not an easy feat. Many who experience depression for the first time do not realize it will not last forever and tend to keep their sadness to themselves and may worry that they are losing their minds.

Some studies show that the teens most likely to kill themselves are those experiencing a clinical depression for the first time. They sometimes believe that they need something to pull them out of it–like a good grade, a new boyfriend, or girlfriend–and when that doesn't happen, they feel worse. Depression can create a psychic pain that becomes unbearable, just as a physical pain can become unbearable. They do not want to kill themselves, but kill the pain. If they don't kill themselves, they may reduce the pain through the abuse of alcohol and **drugs,** through self-mutilation, through eating uncontrollably or not eating, through demeaning sexual activities, or through inflicting pain on others, either physically or verbally.

Children manifest different depressive symptoms from those of adults. Children tend to camouflage or mask depression with deliberate behavior such as acting out their feelings through restlessness, temper tantrums, and fighting. Older adolescents may show signs of masked depression, such as driving recklessly, engaging in risky sexual behavior, as well as the classic adult symptoms–disturbed sleeping habits, change in appetite, and inability to concentrate.

Q & A

Question: What is the link between mental health and suicide?

Answer: Up to 90 percent of people who die by suicide are suffering from some form of mental-health issue—depression, substance abuse, or other diagnosable disorders. Often, this is not determined until after death because many of these people are never detected, assessed, or diagnosed. While the presence of a mental-health issue is strongly associated with suicide, it is important to note that most people with a mental-health issue do not die by suicide, and a mental-health issue does not singularly cause suicide.

Where there is hope, there is life–something to live for and what is generally known as a lifeline. When life has meaning, it is worth living. Having a lifeline gives meaning, gives hope. It can be thought of as a rope to which a drowning person can hang onto as they are engulfed in sorrow. When an individual is submerged in hopelessness, disappointment, disillusionment, despair, emotional isolation, feeling bitter and aching inside, he or she is in search of a lifeline because most people do not want to put an end to turmoil by completing suicide. Most people want to live. In *The Enigma of Suicide,* author George Howe Colt explains that adolescents who depend on others for a sense of self-worth may find a reason to live in someone. They put all their eggs in one basket—a sport, a grade, a person—and it becomes major in their lives. In other words, living is dependent on something and can sometimes be a boyfriend or girlfriend. If the adolescent has no other sources of self-esteem, the relationship becomes tremendously overvalued and becomes the foundation of the person's life, according to some researchers. If good grades are your only form of self-esteem and the only thing that keeps you going, one F can be devastating.

Q & A

Question: If a person is suicidal, does that mean he or she will always be suicidal?

Answer: If a person is suicidal, he or she is looking for a way to end the pain. It does not mean the person wants to die. If he or she gets help, thoughts of suicide will eventually go away. Many people who have been suicidal, after receiving help, go on to live rewarding and meaningful lives.

For many years, there was very little knowledge of the psychological characteristics of young people between the ages of 10 and 24 who took their own lives. Through psychological autopsies, which are studies examining the suicide victim's surroundings—family, friends—some answers have emerged. These studies found that up to 90 percent of adolescent suicide completers have a diagnosable mental disorder at the time of their death. According to *Adolescent Suicide,* Alan Berman and his coauthors indicated that there is evidence that seriously suicidal youth display antisocial behavior or **conduct disorders** more so than other mental disorders. Other studies have indicated a large proportion of young male suicides have been found to have a combination of depression and antisocial or aggressive behaviors, often complicated by drug or alcohol abuse.

The relationship between depression and suicide is not simple. Being young and depressed does not mean you will become suicidal. The vast majority of depressed teens are not suicidal. Usually, suicidality sets in when depression is associated with a deficit in coping skills, and there is substance abuse, hopelessness, and feelings of self-worthlessness.

TEENS SPEAK

I Tried to Stop the Pain

I used to enjoy waking up to the sound of the birds on a lovely spring morning. The sound, that used to be a delight, makes anxiety run through my body with the thought that now, against my will, I have to get up and face another day of my difficult life. In the morning my pain is so excruciating, that with the amount of weight I put on my crutch, I am surprised I don't fall over. I begin to walk up the stairs to the shower as I am holding back all my tears, praying for God to take my pain away, doing everything I can to just try and tough it out.

It all started in the fall of 2006. I was working as a waitress at the local pool hall when I was recovering from a breakup with my boyfriend. I was going through so much emotional agony during work and because I couldn't take it any more, I wanted to just leave. I decided to make myself sick. Knowing I couldn't drink on the job, I went to the medicine cabinet and grabbed a bunch of pills. During my break, I took more than 40 pills. Going through my head was the thought that this would make me so sick that not only would I be out of work for a couple of days, but I also wouldn't have the energy to dwell on the breakup.

Within the next 20 minutes, I could feel the pills doing their job. I began to throw up, over and over again. It started out all liquid and continued with blood as I was throwing up the lining of my stomach. I passed out on the bathroom floor, and next thing I knew I was on a stretcher being transported to the hospital. The only thing I could remember from the hospital was that everything was blurry and bright. They released me, saying that I just had a panic attack, not knowing that I took any pills, which I neglected to tell them because I was ashamed. At home, I was vomiting every five minutes and I could barely focus on anything. I knew I was so messed up that I needed to go back to the hospital. Everything after that was history.

I woke up, having no clue where I was, about two weeks later. I tried moving my body, but I realized I had multiple cords attach to me and an odd pain in my stomach. I saw my mom and dad around my bed with tears in their eyes. I asked where I was and how I got there. My parents proceeded to tell me that I had had a liver transplant. The pills that I took sat in my liver so long they killed everything. I developed bed sores on my backside which were huge, painful, bleeding blisters. I suffered from bruising and pain all over my body. I gained 72 pounds due to fluid retention. But most of all, I realized what the word *family* meant. My dad was at the hospital every day but one out of the whole month and a half that I was in there. This was, what I thought, the most difficult thing I had ever been through, until I learned that I might not ever be able to walk again.

I have not been able to walk without a crutch for almost two years. My body is nothing but scars, immobility, and nonstop pain. I was bitter at the world for a long time because I hated myself for what I did, but everything changed when a friend came along and invited me to church. I had always been very hesitant about church because I didn't like worship and I never really understood the Bible, but when I walked into this church, I felt like I was in a room filled with family. I'm not bitter anymore. The best thing that ever happened to me was getting a new liver, but the most important thing was realizing that I needed faith to make it through the difficulties in life.

DID YOU KNOW?

Bipolar Disorder and Suicide

Bipolar affective disorder is associated with the highest completed suicide rate of any mental disorder.

Source: Kay Redfield Jamison, 1999.

Treatment

Treatment for depression depends on how severe the symptoms are as well as the age of the person suffering from depression. Youths who exhibit symptoms of depression should be referred to mental-health professionals who specialize in treating children and teenagers. Although some young people may think depression will last forever, it might not be the case, and there is hope. Major depressive episodes in adolescents usually last from four to nine months. Often, significant relief comes shortly after treatment begins. Treatment of major depression, using **medication** and psychotherapy, can be effective for children as well as for adults.

BIPOLAR DISORDER AND SUICIDE

Children or teens with bipolar disorder, also called manic-depressive disorder, exhibit serious mood swings. An individual with bipolar disorder can have moods that go up (mania) and down (depression) very quickly, even in one day. The first signs of bipolar disorder are severe moodiness, unhappiness, or other symptoms of depression. Bipolar disorder in children is very often difficult to diagnose, and the symptoms often resemble those of other conditions such as hyperactivity in boys and premenstrual syndrome in girls. Experts used to believe that bipolar disorder was rare in children but now recognize that bipolar disorder presents itself differently in children than in adults.

Depression symptoms of bipolar disorder include:

- continuous sad or irritable mood
- loss of interest in activities a child once enjoyed, such as hobbies, sports, games, or friends
- significant changes in appetite or body weight (weight loss or weight gain)

- sleeping too much or too little or having problems falling asleep
- slow or agitated body movements or restlessness
- no energy or loss of energy
- inappropriate feelings of guilt or worthlessness
- difficulty concentrating
- recurrent thoughts or talks of death or suicide

Mania symptoms of bipolar disorder include:

- severe changes in mood from being extremely irritable or sad to overly silly and elated
- too much energy, such as the ability to keep going without tiring while the child's peers are tiring
- decreased need to sleep, such as going for days with very little or no sleep and not being tired
- talking too much or too fast, changing topics too quickly, and not allowing interruptions
- increased distraction and constantly moving from one thing to another
- a belief in unrealistic abilities or powers
- increased sexual thoughts, feelings, activity, and use of sexual language
- increased obsession with reaching goals or becoming involved in too many activities

Multiple suicide attempts are common among bipolar patients, and research suggests that anywhere from 25 to 50 percent of patients with bipolar disorder have attempted suicide and between 10 and 15 percent eventually die by suicide, especially if it goes untreated. The challenge with this disorder is that the symptoms can resemble or co-occur with those of other common childhood-onset mental disorders. For instance, bipolar disorder may be mistaken for normal emotions and behaviors of children and adolescents. It can also be mistaken for symptoms of trauma or abuse, as well as symptoms of drug use. For example, user of cocaine when a person is under the influence can look like mania, exhibiting the excessive talking, high energy, and little need for sleep.

In adults with bipolar disorder, mood swings usually occur over weeks or even months. In children, cycles or mood swings usually occur more rapidly, sometimes within the same day (referred to as rapid cycling). Frequently, children with bipolar disorder have difficulty getting it together in the morning but then have intense energy later in the day. Often, the mood shifts are continuous, rarely returning to a normal mood between extremes. Sometimes elements of depression and mania or hypomania may be present at the same time, a situation known as a mixed state. These rapid and severe mood changes may make children appear constantly irritable, and they can significantly interfere with their ability to function at school, at home, and with peers.

More specifically, during a manic episode, an adolescent may have high energy and feel extremely happy. This adolescent may need less sleep and may talk on and on, nonstop. He or she may be aggressive and get into fights. The fights may cause either suspension, detention, or an arrest. In addition, for girls, a manic episode could lead to an unwanted teen pregnancy or a sexually transmitted disease from having unsafe sex. During a depressive episode or a down swing of the cycle, an adolescent can be withdrawn or quiet, do poorly in school, and no longer participate in activities once enjoyed, such as dropping out of the basketball team or the drama club. During a down swing, they may cry a lot, sleep too much, and have feelings of self-worthlessness. They may also make threats of suicide.

Treatment
The first line of treatment is to stabilize the child's mood. Doctors often prescribe mood stabilizers such as lithium or Depakote. They also treat sleep disturbances and psychotic symptoms if any are present. Once the

---

DID YOU KNOW?

Stimulants and Anxiety

Caffeine and other stimulants can produce certain forms of anxiety.

It is important to evaluate your use of caffeine and other stimulants.

Source: Massachusetts General Hospital, School Psychiatry Program and MADI Resource Center, 2006.

child is stable, therapy that helps him or her understand the nature of the illness and how it affects his or her emotions; behavior is a critical component of a comprehensive treatment plan.

ANXIETY DISORDERS

These mental disorders are caused by biological changes in the brain, which are the result of fears that are out of control. This type of disorder causes one to feel frightened and uneasy during situations in which others nearby would not experience the same feelings. **Anxiety disorders** in children who do not want to go to school or do not want to engage in conversations or playtime may cause them later in life to use drugs or alcohol to make them feel less anxious. There are five common anxiety disorders.

Panic Attack

A panic disorder results in sudden feelings of terror that strike repeatedly and without warning and sometimes for no apparent reason. Physical symptoms include chest pain, sweating, trembling or shaking, shortness of breath, heart palpitations, abdominal discomfort, dizziness, feelings of unreality, chills and hot flashes, and fear of dying. Children and adolescents with this disorder may experience unrealistic worry, self-consciousness, and tension.

Obsessive-compulsive disorder (OCD)

OCD is described as repeated, intrusive, and unwanted thoughts (obsessions) that cause anxiety or stress and/or rituals that seem impossible to control (compulsions). Adolescents may be aware that their symptoms do not make sense and are excessive, but younger children may be distressed only when they are prevented from carrying out their compulsive habits. Compulsive behaviors often include counting, arranging, and rearranging objects, or excessive hand washing. The obsessions or compulsions cause distress, take time out the day, and interfere with the person's normal routine or functioning.

Post-traumatic stress disorder (PTSD)

PTSD comes from being exposed to a traumatic event such as physical or emotional abuse; natural disasters like a hurricane or tornado or flood; witnessing extreme violence; or being a victim of violence such as being robbed. Symptoms include nightmares; flashbacks; the numbing of emotions; depression; feeling angry, irritable, and distracted; and being easily startled or frightened.

Phobias

Two types of phobias have been identified—specific phobias and social phobias, or social anxiety disorder. A specific phobia is a disabling and irrational fear of something that actually poses little or no actual danger. Examples of specific phobias would be a fear of flying, heights, animals, receiving an injection, or seeing blood. The fear leads to avoidance of these situations and can cause extreme feelings of terror, dread, and panic, which can substantially restrict a person's life.

Social phobias involve fear of certain social situations such as being exposed to unfamiliar people or being exposed to a particular gender. Common symptoms for children and adolescents with social phobias are hypersensitivity to criticism, difficulty being assertive, and low self-esteem.

Generalized anxiety disorder

Generalized anxiety disorder is a chronic, exaggerated worry about everyday, routine life events and activities, which lasts at least six months. People with this disorder find it difficult to control the worry. Children and adolescents with this disorder usually anticipate the worst and often complain of fatigue, tension, headaches, and nausea.

TREATMENT

Effective treatments for anxiety disorders include medication, specific forms of psychotherapy (known as behavioral therapy and cognitive-behavioral therapy), family therapy, or a combination of these. Cognitive-behavioral treatment involves the young person's learning to deal with his or her fears by modifying the way he or she thinks and behaves by practicing new behaviors. There are other more specific treatments for each anxiety disorder depending on the context of the disorder.

A panic disorder is one of the most treatable of all the anxiety disorders, responding in most cases to certain kinds of medication or certain kinds of cognitive psychotherapy, which help change thinking patterns that lead to fear and anxiety. OCD usually responds well to treatment with certain medications and/or exposure-based psycho-therapy, in which people face situations that cause fear or anxiety and become less sensitive (desensitized) to them. PTSD is often accom-panied by depression, substance abuse, or one or more of the other anxiety disorders. Certain kinds of medication and certain kinds of psychotherapy usually treat the symptoms of PTSD very effectively. Phobias can also be treated with certain kinds of psychotherapy or medications. Generalized anxiety disorder is commonly treated with medication or cognitive-behavioral therapy, but co-occurring condi-tions, or those conditions such as alcohol abuse or depression that accompany the anxiety, must also be treated using the appropriate therapies.

According to the National Institute of Mental Health, medica-tion will not cure anxiety disorders, but it can keep them under control while the person receives psychotherapy. Medication must be prescribed by physicians, usually psychiatrists, who can either offer psychotherapy themselves or work as a team with psycholo-gists, social workers, or counselors who provide psychotherapy. The principal medications used for anxiety disorders are antidepressants, antianxiety drugs, and beta-blockers to control some of the physical symptoms. With proper treatment, many people with anxiety disor-ders can lead normal, fulfilling lives.

Antianxiety Drugs

High-potency benzodiazepines combat anxiety and have few side effects other than drowsiness. Because people can get used to them and may need higher and higher doses to get the same effect, ben-zodiazepines are generally prescribed for short periods of time, espe-cially for people who have abused drugs or alcohol and who become dependent on medication easily. One exception to this rule is that people with panic disorder can take benzodiazepines for up to a year or in some cases longer without harm.

One drug that is used for social phobia and generalized anxiety disorder is clonazepam (Klonopin). Lorazepam (Ativan) is helpful for panic disorder, and alprazolam (Xanax) is useful for both panic dis-order and generalized anxiety disorder.

Some people experience withdrawal symptoms if they stop taking benzodiazepines abruptly instead of tapering off, and anxiety can return once the medication is stopped. These potential problems have led some physicians to shy away from using these drugs or to use them in inadequate doses.

Buspirone (Buspar) is a newer antianxiety medication used to treat generalized anxiety disorder. Possible side effects include dizziness, headaches, and nausea. Unlike benzodiazepines, buspirone must be taken consistently for at least two weeks to achieve an antianxiety effect.

The **selective serotonin reuptake inhibitors (SSRI)**, which are often referred to as antidepressants, are also quite effective in treating certain kinds of anxiety disorders, including panic disorder and OCD. These medications include fluoxetine (Prozac), paroxetine (Paxil and others), sertraline (Zoloft and others), and others.

Helpful hints for managing anxiety include relaxation techniques such as deep breathing—breathing in deeply and out slowly, counting to 10, or visualizing a soothing place such as the water on a beach. Relaxing can help people manage their symptoms and give a sense of control over the body. Getting to school in the morning or preparing for bed in the evening may be complicated by fears and anxieties. Anticipating and planning for these transition times may be helpful.

In conclusion, if a mental illness is contributing to suicidal behavior, the illness needs to be managed—preferably through treatment. If treatment is not available, engaging in self-support techniques can help or consulting an adult or someone from your school who could help you obtain treatment. In essence, no one really knows why people kill themselves. Experts can only make educated guesses from what research reveals. We do know that mental illnesses contribute to the cause of suicide in many cases, but not all cases. For example, people can be diagnosed with bipolar disorder and live very successful lives—or may ultimately kill themselves because of the inability to get the proper treatment needed. Thus, it is important for people with a mental disorder that might lead to suicide to get treated and comply with the treatment.

See also: Biology of Suicidal Behavior; Suicide Prevention

■ MINORITIES AND SUICIDE

See: Ethnicity and Suicide; Suicide and the Gay, Lesbian, Bisexual, and Transgender Communities

Suicide Rates Among Young People

Ages 10-14

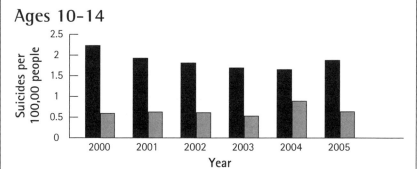

Ages 15-19

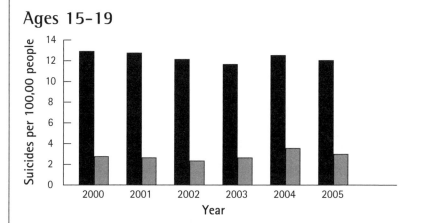

Ages 20-24

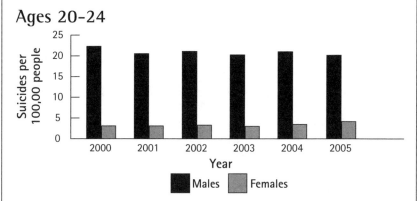

■ Males ■ Females

In 2005, suicide was the third-leading cause of death among children and young adults aged 10 to 24 years in the United States.

Source: Centers for Disease Control and Prevention, National Vital Statistics System, www.cdc.gov, 2006.

■ NATIVE AMERICANS

See: Ethnicity and Suicide

■ PREVALENCE AND EPIDEMIOLOGY

The occurrence of suicides and the factors that affect the increase or decrease of suicides among young adults. How prevalent is suicide, and why does it occur?

As indicated by the data in the charts, there is an increase shown in suicides among females from 2003 to 2004 in the younger age categories and an increase among males between ages 15 and 19. There is also an increase shown from 2004 to 2005 for males ages 10 to 14. And in 2005, suicide was reported to be the third-leading cause of death among all young people over 10.

CONTRIBUTING FACTORS

A suicide can be precipitated, or triggered, when life no longer has meaning and loses its purpose or when life becomes difficult. However, in order to understand suicide, experts try to determine which difficulties in life are most dangerous or can become **triggers** for suicide. What becomes difficult for one person may not be difficult for another.

In ancient Roman culture, the primary reasons for suicide were shame, grief, and despair. In modern Europe, when suicides were studied, it was concluded that insanity and alcoholism were the primary reasons for suicide, followed by incurable diseases and disappointed love. What then are the contributing factors to suicide among teens in the 21st century? What leads to negative emotions? Recent studies tell us family conflicts, tension in relationships (especially for girls), low self-esteem, and anxiety are symptoms that could lead to distorted thinking—thinking that leads to distorted perceptions that get in the way of happiness and causes hopelessness and misery.

In 2004, there were substantial increases in rates of substance use and abuse, according to the Centers for Disease Control's Morbidity and Mortality Weekly Report. The number of **drug**-induced deaths had increased more than 50 percent in 2004 from 1999. Drug-induced deaths were primarily caused by overdoses of illegal drugs and legal drugs taken for nonmedical reasons, poisoning from legal drugs taken in error or at the wrong dose, and poisoning from other substances such as alcohol, pesticides, or carbon monoxide. Changes in rates of substance use and abuse could be a contributing factor.

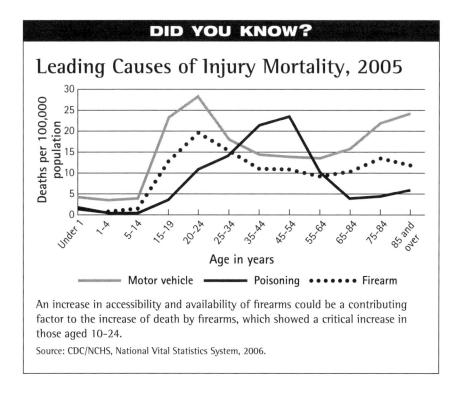

DID YOU KNOW?

Leading Causes of Injury Mortality, 2005

Motor vehicle ▬▬▬ Poisoning •••••• Firearm

An increase in accessibility and availability of firearms could be a contributing factor to the increase of death by firearms, which showed a critical increase in those aged 10-24.

Source: CDC/NCHS, National Vital Statistics System, 2006.

SUICIDES ARE A MATTER OF TIMING

One of the myths common to suicides is that the rate increases during the winter holidays—mainly December. However, December has the fewest suicides per day, with an increase in suicides in the spring or between March and September according to some studies. A study was conducted by the CDC in 2001 on violent deaths in middle, junior, and senior high schools in the United States during the period 1992–99. The results of the study showed that student homicide events were usually highest near the start of the fall and spring semesters, and suicide events were highest during the spring semester.

METHODS OF SUICIDE

The three most common methods for completed suicides are firearm, hanging/suffocation, and poisoning. For adolescents, the methods are usually those that can be found in the home, as one study reports that 70 percent of completers killed themselves at home and 22 percent outdoors. However, the methods used by children and teens to complete suicide changed significantly over the last decade. The use of firearms decreased substantially, and hanging increased between the ages of 10 and 14 and also increased slightly for ages 15 to 19.

NONFATAL SELF-INFLICTED INJURY

The level and nature of the problem of suicide extends to suicidal behavior and suicide attempts. There is one suicide for every 25

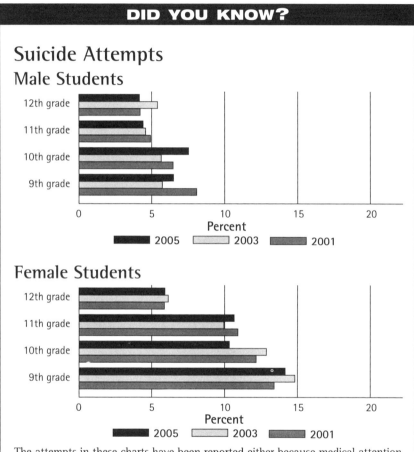

DID YOU KNOW?

Suicide Attempts
Male Students

Male Students chart: grades 12th, 11th, 10th, 9th. Bars for 2005, 2003, 2001. X-axis: Percent, 0 to 20.

Female Students

Female Students chart: grades 12th, 11th, 10th, 9th. Bars for 2005, 2003, 2001. X-axis: Percent, 0 to 20.

The attempts in these charts have been reported either because medical attention was needed or they occurred in hospitals, schools, or jails. Attempts that do not require medical attention, or perhaps happened in the home, rarely get reported. Studies suggest that the majority of attempts go unreported, according to what students have revealed when surveyed. Therefore, there are many more suicide attempts than the rates indicate.

Source: National Center for Injury Prevention and Control, 2006.

attempted suicides across the life span. There is one suicide for every 100–200 attempts for young adults age 15–24. In 2005, 16.9 percent of U.S. high school students reported that they had seriously considered attempting suicide, and more than 8 percent of students reported that they had actually attempted suicide one or more times during the same period. The chart on page 83 is a more accurate view of suicide attempts across the United States.

See also: Alcohol, Drugs, and Suicide; Suicide Prevention

FURTHER READINGS

Berman, Alan, David Jobes, and Morton Silverman. *Adolescent Suicide: Assessment and Intervention.* New York: Gilford Press, 2002.

Collins, Christine, Ph.D., and Ron Salomon, M.D. *Suicide.* New York: Chelsea House, 2007.

Salomon, Ron. *Suicide.* New York: Chelsea House, 2007.

■ PREVENTION

See: American Foundation for Suicide Prevention; Suicide Prevention

■ RISK AND PROTECTIVE FACTORS FOR SUICIDE

Risk factors are any circumstances in teenagers' lives that may increase their chances of engaging in suicidal behavior, such as talking about suicide, making suicidal gestures, or engaging in destructive behavior. Therefore, many factors contribute to the risk of becoming suicidal, attempting suicide, or dying by suicide. What happens is that the risk factors begin lining up and can cause one to think that death is an option. There are several types of risk factors: individual, family, school, peer group, and community.

INDIVIDUAL RISK FACTORS

Individual risk factors are those circumstances that pertain to negative attitudes, negative behavior, or negative life **stressors** that develop while growing up, such as demonstrating delinquent beliefs, general delinquency involvement, teen parenthood, aggressiveness, impulsivity, prior attempt, mental health problems, victimization, exposure to violence, learning disabilities, and illegal gun ownership—just to list a few. These are factors that make it likely that youth will engage in risky behaviors that could lead to suicidal thoughts or gestures.

FAMILY RISK FACTORS

Family risk factors can develop when there is a **family history** of problem behavior that includes criminal behavior committed by the parents, child abuse, family violence, family transition such as divorce, and poor family bonding, as well as poor parental supervision. Children have no control over what goes on in the family, and many are affected by negative behaviors performed by the parents. If parents fail to set good standards for their teen's behavior, it increases the likelihood that the teen will engage in street behavior such as substance abuse, gang activity, or other delinquent behavior.

SCHOOL RISK FACTORS

School risk factors include having low academic grades or achievement, a negative attitude toward school with no real commitment, truancy record that could lead to suspension or suspension in general, dropping out of school with no real goals for the future, and an inadequate school climate with poorly organized teachers who give the students negative labels. School is a major part of adolescence life. Teens spend most of their day in school. If school is making a teen unhappy, it means most of his or her day is spent in misery. This could lead to a snowball effect causing the student to engage in delinquent behavior just for kicks, getting in trouble with the law because of the truancy record, or causing family conflicts because the parents want the teen to do better in school.

Q & A

Question: If depressed and suicidal people seem to feel better, does this mean they won't take their own lives?

Answer: Sometimes people who are severely depressed and contemplating suicide don't have the energy to carry it out. However, as the disease begins to rescind and they begin to feel better, they may regain some of their energy but will still have feelings of hopelessness, and anxiety can sometimes set in. The anxiousness can cause a risk for suicide or a suicide attempt coupled by the renewed energy. There is also another theory that people give in to the anguished feelings caused by the **depression** or disease because they cannot fight it anymore. This releases some of their anxiety because they have made a decision to end it all, which makes them appear calmer, as though they are feeling better. If a person seems better, he or she may indeed be feeling better and is not considering suicide. However, the only way to determine if a person who seems to be feeling better is actually better or worse is to have a direct and open discussion about suicide more than once.

PEER GROUP RISK FACTORS

Peers have a large influence on youth. If there is not a strong family influence, the influence of peers can be overpowering. How the friends act, think, and feel becomes contagious. Sometimes there is a positive effect, but when there is a negative effect with poor influences, peers become a risk factor. If the peers engage in alcohol, tobacco or **drug** use, that is a negative influence. If the teen is exposed to similar abuse of alcohol, tobacco, and drugs in the home, another negative influence may determine whether or not he or she is able to identify with the peers. Teens are more likely to engage in deviant behaviors if they are part of a family that stresses and promotes deviant lifestyles.

Another note of interest is that most often teens relate better to peers. Parents tend to dominate, and school tends to discipline and dictate, while peers allow a teen to assert himself or herself. Therefore, friends become very important in a young adult's life. Not only are bad influences from peers a risk factor, but also peers can be a source of humiliation and harassment. While peers for the most part are supportive, some teens will find a few peers that bully and make fun of others. This becomes painful to the individual being bullied or harassed, and an action such as this has lead to suicidal behavior, if not death by suicide. As mentioned in a previous chapter, Joshua, age 15, took his own life after being constantly harassed at school for his differences.

COMMUNITY RISK FACTORS

Certain communities or neighborhoods where children grow up can disrupt the flow of a good upbringing and put the children at a disadvantage. For instance, if a community offers easy access to alcohol, tobacco, and other drugs in the neighborhood, teens will be tempted to engage. Communities can be sites for bad behavior if there is high crime, availability of firearms, poverty, vacant buildings and lots, and poor schools. Children can also witness violent events and can become fearful living in their own neighborhood. This fear can cause them to become a part of the violence to protect themselves by joining a gang or acquiring a gun. Children begin learning that violence is acceptable behavior that is valued and normal.

BIOPSYCHOSOCIAL CHARACTERISTICS

The other risk factor that is very important is the biopsychosocial factor—a combination of biological, psychological, and social risk factors. This risk factor encompasses biology, such as mental disorders that are based on chemical imbalances in the brain; psychology, such as chronic hopelessness, aggressiveness, and impulsivity, all of which deal with the emotions; and social factors, which deal with the environment or daily surroundings, such as a family history of alcoholism, trauma, or abuse.

ASSESSING RISK FACTORS

Risk factors for suicide generally function cumulatively or add up to a number of risk factors at one time. The more risk factors, the greater the likelihood that a youth will engage in suicidal behavior. With hopelessness being the key risk factor, depression, family problems, school issues, and friends with bad behavior all add up. If several risk factors affect a teen's life at the same time, protective factors need to set in.

Q & A

Question: Is it possible to stop someone from killing herself if she is convinced she wants to die?

Answer: If people in a suicidal crisis get the help they need, they will probably never be suicidal again. According to the long research conducted by the QPR Institute in Spokane, Washington, suicide is the most preventable death because most victims really do not want to die; they just want the pain to go away.

PROTECTIVE FACTORS

Protective factors are those that help guard an individual from becoming suicidal. They act as safeguards. Protective factors operate in several ways: (1) They serve as a buffer to cushion the affects of the negative circumstances going on around them; (2) they can interrupt the process of a negative risk factor that is damaging in teen life by decreasing the effects such as removing an alcoholic and abusive parent from the house; and (3) they can prevent the initial occurrence of a risk factor by building strong morals in the household and insuring that the family has a solid spiritual belief system that can offer hope in times of stress.

Individual factors

Individual protective factors develop when a person has a positive temperament, which is exactly opposite of the individual risk factor indicating a constant negative attitude. Having a positive attitude toward your daily routine builds resiliency. When a person stays connected to his or her surroundings, it affords structure and discipline. Being committed to school, attached to the family, and involved in the community builds a strong foundation that keeps an individual grounded with a healthy sense of self.

Family

Quality relationships with parents and an attachment to family helps serve as a buffer from stresses. Good family support develops when a family is stable and there is open communication with family members.

Fact Or Fiction?

Confronting a person about suicide will only make them angry and increase the risk of suicide.

The Facts: Asking someone directly about suicidal intent lowers anxiety and opens up the line of communication. It also lowers the risk of an impulsive suicide.

Bullying, depression, and suicide

Bullying is defined as engaging in behaviors such as teasing, being cruel, hurtful and unkind to others, threatening, hitting and stealing that are initiated by one or more students against a victim. Intentional exclusion and causing a student to be socially isolated is another form of bullying. Boys typically engage in the threatening, hitting, and more taunting of a victim, whereas girls are more apt to engage in social isolation by purposely excluding someone or spreading rumors about the victim. Either way, students who are victims of bullying generally suffer from anxiety, insecurity, and low self-esteem.

Clinical depression and suicide are a foreseeable consequence of bullying according to studies in the United States, Korea, Finland, and Great Britain. Victims often fear school and consider school to be an unsafe and unhappy place. One study found as many as 7 percent of America's eighth-graders stay home at least once a month because of bullies.

Students who engage in bullying behaviors seem to have a need to feel powerful and in control. While they get satisfaction from inflicting injury and suffering on others, one study by Riittakerttu Kaltiala-Heino found an increased prevalence of depression and severe suicidal ideation among both those who were bullied and those who were bullies. Depression occurred equally frequently among those who were bullied and those who were bullies, but most commonly among those who were both bullied by others and were also bullies themselves.

In a case study of Jared Benjamin High, Jared developed depression from bullying at school as well as an assault by a bully at school. The term used to describe this type of teen suicide is *bullycide,* a suicide caused by bullying. When 13-year-old Jared took his life, his family had the school investigated. As a result, according to Dr. Alan Berman of the American Association of Suicidology, and who conducted a complete investigation, Jared did not exhibit the symptoms of clinical depression prior to the incidents of being bullied. Dr. Berman further concluded that Jared would have not developed depression and the impulse to complete suicide if the bullying had not occurred. A positive attitude toward school and communicating your problem to an adult are protective factors against bullying.

Q & A

Question: Do suicidal people keep their plans to themselves?

Answer: Most suicidal individuals communicate their intent some time during the week preceding their attempt. They communicate either verbally or make suicidal gestures. Gestures include actions that are taken to resemble an attempt while not being fully committed to die yet. Examples include taking too many pills but yet not enough to die, or planning to die by practicing tying a knot in the rope to be used to hang oneself.

Peer factors

Peers can serve as a buffer. This is especially true when a teen is suffering from negative effects from home and there is involvement with positive peer group activities and norms.

Community factors

A community that has good resources such as activities for the children and young adults, stable families, schools, and churches influences teenagers' positive traits. It keeps their lives fun-filled and happy. Youth are also more apt to be exposed to good adult role models other than their parents when communities have informal sources of adult supervision and neighborhoods and when city services are functioning.

Good human self-worth

Good self-image, self-esteem, and self-confidence all contribute to one's mental well-being and attitude toward life and work as protective factors. Having good problem-solving skills and good social support from family and friends help strengthen one's social network. A good emotional relationship with at least one person and positive school experience helps as well.

FURTHER READINGS

Collins, Christine, Ph.D., and Ron Salomon, M.D. *Suicide.* New York: Chelsea House, 2007.

Grollman, Earl A. *Suicide: Prevention, Intervention, Postvention.* Boston: Beacon Press, 1988.

See also: Culture and Suicide; Suicide Prevention

■ RUNAWAY TEENAGERS

See: Alcohol, Drugs, and Suicide

■ SELF-INJURIOUS BEHAVIOR

Behavior in which a person does harm to himself or herself. *Self-injury, self-harm, self-inflicted violence,* or *self-directed violence* are all terms used to describe a deliberate injury inflicted on one's own body without suicidal intent. It is estimated that 1 to 2 million people in the United States purposely bruise and cut various parts of their bodies. However, this estimate represents only those cases that are reported, either because the person sought help for the behavior or because the infliction needed medical attention. The majority of the time, medical attention is not needed or the case is dismissed as an accident. Also, many self-injurers are very self-conscious of their wounds and go to great lengths to conceal their behavior from others. The act is usually carried out in private. People may offer alternative explanations for their injuries or conceal their scars with clothing. When this behavior is exhibited by young people who also threaten suicide, the condition is called **adolescent suicide syndrome.**

Both males and females may engage in self-injurious behavior and often begin in early adolescence. This behavior peaks between the ages of 18 and 24 and decreases during the 30s and 40s. There are some rare cases in which the behavior begins in childhood and continues into middle age.

THE PURPOSE OF SELF-INJURIOUS BEHAVIOR

Self-harmers are often mistaken as suicidal, but research has shown that the majority of the cases are nonfatal. These self-inflictions are not to be thought of as attempted suicides. Based on these studies, people, mostly children and young adults, engage in self-injurious behaviors to experience a relief from emotional pain. They can feel physical pain, and this removes attention from internal emotional agony they are experiencing. Adolescents are particularly vulnerable as they face many difficult and inherently stressful challenges as they grow and develop. It is a time of uncertainty as they go through an adolescent identity crisis—trying to figure out what it means to be an adult. The body as well as the mind goes through profound changes and disruptions. Puberty is in its final stages, and sexual development is setting in. They are experiencing accelerated growth as they grow taller and larger. Hormones are being released that contribute to their flow of energy. They are no longer carefree kids, and they now struggle with the need of peer acceptance and the possibility of making new friends.

Self-harm is primarily a coping strategy. This behavior can be triggered by a traumatic event such as witnessing a violent act at a young age that is difficult to overcome. The event can create negative thoughts such as "I am a failure" and negative feelings such as rage and misery.

Without the proper coping skills or lack of knowledge on how to handle the thoughts and feelings, tension and anxiety can set in. As the tension builds, adolescents begin to zone out or dissociate. They are looking for an escape and will hurt the body. According to a 2002 article by Lisa Ferentz, founder and president of the Advanced Psychotherapy Training and Education, Inc.:

> The dissociative process allows teenagers to detach from their own bodies, their environment and their behavior. As the body is injured, they immediately experience positive effects. The negative thoughts and feelings are forgotten and a fleeting sense of control is reclaimed. Perhaps, most importantly, the body responds to the trauma of injury by releasing **endorphins**: naturally occurring opiates. The release of endorphins allows the teenager to feel "high," "euphoric" and "relieved." The shock of seeing blood helps some teenagers feel "alive and real." Unfortunately, the positive effects are always followed by negative outcomes, including a loss of control, a feeling of failure, shame and guilt, **depression** and self-hatred. Some adolescents have no conscious memory of hurting themselves and are actually frightened when they discover a wound. Others report that they can "watch themselves" engage in self-harm, but they feel "powerless" to stop the process. These negative outcomes leave the teen emotionally vulnerable and primed to be triggered by the next "threatening" event. This helps to explain the repetitive or cyclical nature of self-injurious behavior.

As noted earlier, self-injurious behavior is not considered suicidal. Those who engage in self-injurious behaviors are most likely feeling a lot of internal pain and may be experiencing symptoms of anxiety or depression. Because there is a strong link between suicidality and depression, however, it is important for concerned others to invite open communication about self-injury and suicidality.

TYPES OF SELF-INJURIOUS BEHAVIOR

Self-injury is manifested in several forms, most commonly cutting, scraping, burning, biting, or hitting. The most common type is cutting and slashing. However, many teens do it in a variety of ways such as burning the skin, head banging, picking old wounds, peeling the skin, deep biting, severe skin scratching, nail and cuticle biting, pulling hair, bone breaking, and swallowing sharp objects. The most targeted parts of the body are the arms.

It is not uncommon for young adults who hurt themselves to engage in other forms of destructive behavior such as reckless driving, shoplifting, sexual promiscuity or unprotected sex, substance abuse, and eating-disordered behaviors. An individual who engages in self-harm is desperately trying to cope with overwhelming feelings and thoughts. Self-inflicted violence is meant to soothe, alleviate anxiety, and increase a sense of power and control. Ironically, as the behavior escalates, it actually worsens feelings of disempowerment, alienation, and helplessness.

Self-destructive behaviors are not to be confused with body piercing or tattoos that are sought for the purpose creating art on the body. However, teenagers who allow piercing to become infected and then pick at the wounds or secretly pierce or tattoo their own bodies to relieve anxiety or "feel better" are engaging in self-injury.

There are two different reasons that individuals may harm themselves: *hyperstress* and *dissociation.* Hyperstress occurs when a person is hypersensitive and overwhelmed. A great many thoughts may be revolving within his or her mind, becoming confused and entangled. The person may be upset and tearful, or angry and destructive; he or she may well experience physical symptoms such as nausea or a racing heart. He or she may become triggered, making the decision to stop the overwhelming feelings by resorting to self-injury. A **trigger** is an event that upsets and disturbs a person; it could be an internal event within the mind or an external event that affects the person. Triggers can make a person feel a great deal worse, and there is a feeling of panic and a need to directly and immediately end the distress—hence self-harm. Self-injury can have an immediate soothing effect, slowing the mind down, calming the breathing and heart rate, and enabling the person to cope, regain control, and continue to function.

On the other hand, a person can experience dissociation and be detached from life, detached from their emotions and from their body, feeling numb. They may feel separate from reality and may behave without being aware of what they are doing. People suffering trauma or abuse may learn to dissociate themselves from what is happening. They may find that dissociation becomes an automatic response to stressful situations. When in a dissociated frame of mind, a trigger is

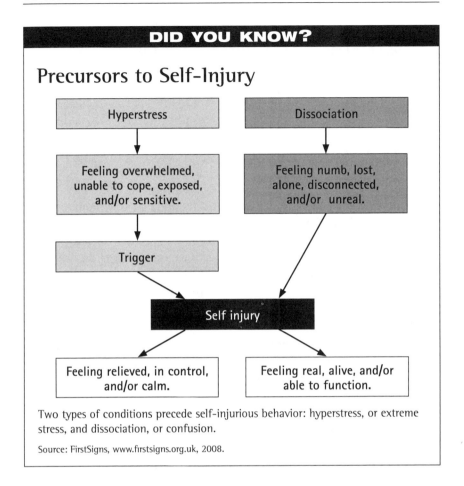

DID YOU KNOW?

Precursors to Self-Injury

Hyperstress → Feeling overwhelmed, unable to cope, exposed, and/or sensitive.

Dissociation → Feeling numb, lost, alone, disconnected, and/or unreal.

Trigger

Self injury

Feeling relieved, in control, and/or calm.

Feeling real, alive, and/or able to function.

Two types of conditions precede self-injurious behavior: hyperstress, or extreme stress, and dissociation, or confusion.

Source: FirstSigns, www.firstsigns.org.uk, 2008.

not present. Individuals recognize the need to get control of themselves and experience a desire to feel real again and act in a way that will create a sensation—and for this reason engage in self-harm.

Gender differences

According to recent studies, four times as many females as males have direct experience of self-harm. The World Health Organization found the female rate of self-injury exceeded that of males, with the highest rate among females in the 15–24 age group and the highest rate among males in the 12–34 age group. However, when a study was done on 428 homeless and runaway youth age 16 to 19, 72 percent of males and 66 percent of females reported a past history of self-mutilation.

Furthermore, the Mental Health Foundation reports that one must be aware that males can be just as susceptible to self-injurious behavior but engage in different forms of self-harm such as hitting and punching themselves or breaking bones, which may be easier to hide or be explained as an accident or result of a fight.

There does not appear to be a difference in motivation for self-harm in adolescent males and females. In the Mental Health Foundation's report of the National Inquiry into self-harm among young people, researchers found that those consulted for the inquiry reported a wide range of factors that could trigger self-harm. The most frequent reasons mentioned by youth were:

- being bullied at school
- not getting along with parents
- stress and worry around academic performance and examinations
- parental divorce
- bereavement
- unwanted pregnancy
- experience of abuse in earlier childhood (whether sexual, physical, and/or emotional)
- difficulties associated with sexuality
- problems to do with race, culture, or religion
- low self-esteem
- feelings of being rejected in their lives

LESBIAN, GAY, BISEXUAL, AND TRANSGENDER YOUNG PEOPLE

Recent research from the National Inquiry report indicates that lesbian, gay, bisexual, and transgender young people report higher rates of self-harm than do heterosexual young people. They are two to three times more likely to self-harm. Studies have shown that 72 percent of lesbian, gay, bisexual, and transgender adults reported a regular history of absenteeism at school due to homophobic harassment; 50 percent who had been bullied at school reported they had contemplated self-harm, and 40 percent had self-harmed at least once. Results from a national survey that looked at mental health problems in gay men, lesbians, and bisexuals found that 42 percent of gay men, 43 percent of lesbians, and 49 percent of bisexual men and women have planned or committed acts of self-harm.

The reasons why young lesbian, gay, bisexual, and transgender individuals self-harm are broadly similar to the reasons cited by youth as a whole. Other reports from Great Britain found that young people cited pressure, isolation, not fitting in, anger, and frustration with themselves, **panic attacks,** the need to take control of something, the need to escape, bereavement, and stress caused by examinations and school as reasons why they had self-harmed.

TECHNIQUES TO TRY IF YOU ARE
HAVING SELF-INJURIOUS THOUGHTS

- Remove yourself from the situation you are in, and do something else.
- Talk with someone who is supportive, such as a family member, a school counselor, or a teacher.
- Engage in another activity. Blow bubbles, take a hot or cold shower, squeeze ice, finger paint, or squish Play-doh.
- Go for a brisk walk, or run, punch a pillow, swim, lift weights, or engage in other aerobic activities that require physical exertion.
- Read, listen to music, take a relaxing bath, look at the moon or clouds, open a window to get some fresh air.
- Make a list of activities to engage in that have been helpful in the past when you had the urge to self-injure. Keep this list handy to refer to if you do have the urge to self-injure.
- Keep a journal of your thoughts and urges and write about what helped you not to engage.

Q & A

Question: What kinds of people self-injure, and does it have an impact on their daily lives?

Answer: Self-injurers come from all walks of life and all economic backgrounds, although research shows most come from a middle-class to upper-class background. People who harm themselves can be male or female; straight, gay, or bisexual; high school students or high-school dropouts; rich or poor; from any country in the world. Nearly 50 percent report physical abuse and/or sexual abuse during his or her childhood. Many self-injurers report that they were discouraged from expressing emotions, particularly anger or sadness. The incidence of self-injury is about the same as that of eating disorders, but because it is so highly stigmatized, most people hide their scars, burns, and bruises carefully. They also have excuses ready when someone asks about the scars. It is more difficult to hide an eating disorder.

The guilt and secrecy associated with self-harm most certainly affects self-injurers' daily lives: their relationships, the clothes they wear, their interactions with their friends, and their sense of self-worth. If and when they do tell someone else about their self-harm, the whole issue is frequently taken completely out of their hands, and their previously secretive behavior becomes common knowledge. At any point when they appear even slightly stressed, they are aware that everyone is watching them closely in case they self-harm again. At worst, their self-harm may cause them to be diagnosed with a mental health condition such as borderline personality disorder. Most important, the focus very often remains on the self-harm, not the underlying problems causing them to feel they have no other option but to adopt this self-harming behavior as a coping strategy and keep it a secret.

See also: Gender and Suicide; Mental Illness and Suicide; Stress and Suicide; Suicide and the Gay, Lesbian, Bisexual, and Transgender Communities

FURTHER READING
Bowman, Susan, and Kaye Randall. *See My Pain! Creative Strategies and Activities for Helping Young People Who Self-Injure.* Chapin, S.C.: Youthlight, 2006.
Shapiro, Lawrence E. *Stopping the Pain: A Workbook for Teens Who Cut & Self-Injure.* Oakland, Calif.: Instant Help Books, 2008.

◼ STRESS AND SUICIDE

Psychological and physiological responses to events that upset one's personal balance in some way and the effect on one's suicidal

---

DID YOU KNOW?

Addictions are linked to a stressful lifestyle.

Several addictions are linked to a stressful lifestyle, including over-eating, smoking, drinking, and **drug** abuse. The addictions are used as an escape or a temporary way of "shutting down," but they do not address the root of the stress.

---

behavior or interest in taking one's own life. Stress is simply a reaction to situations, events, or people. For example, failing a test, fighting with a friend, or having an argument with a parent can cause stress. When teens feel tense or stressed by something going on around them, their bodies react by releasing chemicals—such as adrenaline—into the bloodstream. These chemicals cause the body to have more energy in need of an outlet to release the energy—hence tossing and turning and not being able to go to sleep or overeating because the body needs something to do. Generally present are symptoms of anxiety, worry, and withdrawal when we are suffering from stress.

HOW TO TELL IF YOU ARE STRESSED

Signs of stress are sometimes changes in the body, changes in behavior, changes in the emotions, or changes in one's thinking. Below are examples to help identify some of these changes:

Changes in the body

Changes in the way one feels are often indicators that a person is under stress. Signs to watch out for include: nervousness, headaches, stomachaches, restless sleep, overeating or eating too little, and frequent tiredness.

Changes in behavior

Changes in the way a person behaves are also indicators that he or she is under stress. Some behaviors include: increased use of alcohol and drugs, withdrawal from others, increased smoking, nonstop talking, being short-tempered, and fidgeting.

Changes in emotions

A person's emotions can change when a person is under stress. Loneliness, **depression**, confusion and excess worrying, anger and irritability, frequent crying, and feeling hopeless and suicidal are all indicators that someone is under stress and needs help.

Changes in thinking

A person's thinking can also be affected by stress. A person who is under stress might have trouble concentrating; he or she might lack self-confidence, feel worthless; and he or she might make bad decisions.

Once a person knows that he or she is stressed, the person can begin to identify the things that may be causing the stress. Sometimes they will be things one can control, such as getting enough sleep, catching up with schoolwork, or trying to get along better with parents. Then there are things that are beyond one's control such as the death of a parent. It is also important to recognize that no one is in control of all the aspects of life that can create stress. Another **stressor** that can have negative consequences is **anticipatory grief**–grief in expectation of a loved one's death, either because the loved one is suffering from a **terminal illness** or because he or she has hinted about suicide.

Q & A

Question: Can a suicidal person mask his or her depression with happiness?

Answer: Many people suffering from depression can hide their feelings, appearing to be happy. Some are very good at masking—including masking their suicidal thoughts. However, most of the time individuals will give warning signs as to how desperate they are feeling. Their signs may be subtle clues, which is why knowing what the warning signs are is critical. Furthermore, some of the clues may be verbal; for example, they may say something like, "Everyone would be better off without me." Or, "It doesn't matter. I won't be around much longer anyway." Keying in to such phases is important, and the phases should not be dismissed as just "talk."

HOW WE REACT TO STRESS AND PROBLEMS

Stress in life is unavoidable. However, how a person reacts to stress may be regrettable. For example, a person might get angry and scream, shout, throw things, start a fight, or go on a rampage. Or, the person can withdraw by taking a drink, hiding out in a room, or stop talking to everyone.

Aggression and anger get attention. Striking out at someone who a person may think is adding to the problem brings temporary relief. However, aggressive actions, like breaking things, drinking too much, driving recklessly, or swearing at people can cause trouble in the long run. These behaviors do not solve the problem. They only make the problem worse.

Withdrawal can also be destructive. It is normal to want to be left alone at certain times, but if it goes on for a long time, people are without what they need most—friends who can share problems and understanding relatives who may come to one's aid. When people isolate themselves, they end up alone with a problem, and they feel like no one cares. The depression and anger become worse, and they begin to make bad choices instead of healthy ones.

Another reaction to problems and a particularly cruel phenomenon is **pseudocide,** in which a person fakes his or her own death. Usually committed by men, it is a growing occurrence. No one should underestimate the suffering for those left behind by this supremely selfish act. Some people are escaping debts, or violence, or unhappiness, and some are simply seeking to re-create themselves by trying to start anew. Other people are trying to get attention, and still others backfire, resulting in actual suicide. Nonetheless, the effect on families and other survivors is the same as an authentic suicide.

WAYS TO REACT THAT ARE GOOD FOR YOU

If you or someone you know is experiencing problems such as being afraid of failing an exam or moving to another school, you may begin having headaches or an upset stomach. There are a number of things you or your friend can do, such as talking to someone you trust, sharing what is bothering you, and being open about how you feel.

These things do not solve the problem, but they allow you to talk about it so that one can feel better. It is always a good idea to get an adult to help solve a problem. If an adult is not available for you at the moment, try not to engage in "stinking thinking"—or negative thoughts. To help decrease stress, individuals can first learn to change what they say to themselves and the way they think about themselves. Following are a few examples of how a person might turn negative comments into positives ones:

> Negative: To be a worthwhile person, I have to be good at everything.

> Positive: Just being who I am makes me worthwhile.

> Negative: Everyone has to like me, or else I'm not okay.

> Positive: I'm okay just the way I am.

> Negative: I can't help how I feel, and I am feeling miserable.

> Positive: I can make the decision not to feel miserable.

> Negative: I have to worry about everything that could go wrong.

> Positive: I can learn to concentrate on the present moment and relax.

Finding ways to increase one's health also helps decrease stress. Simple ways to do this are:

- Get adequate sleep.
- Exercise more.
- Eat healthy food and less junk food.
- Laugh more and smile more.
- Apply positive attitudes.
- Talk to people you trust.
- Work at managing your time so that you do not fall behind in your schoolwork.
- Make an effort to relax.

Part of life is dealing with stress. When someone is really tense or stressed out, here are a few more things to think about:

- Don't try to please everyone. Leave something for yourself.
- Stress can be an energizer. Control that energy and focus on a positive task.
- Be active. Look for ways you can start to make some plans, or set some goals for yourself.

- Take charge of yourself. You can't control other people's actions, but you can control yours.
- Give yourself a break. Pause and do something for yourself.
- You are not alone. Talk to someone who may be going through the same thing.

AVOID NEGATIVE COPING STRATEGIES

Many teens use negative coping strategies to cope with stress. These are strategies that may temporarily provide stress relief, but in the long term they may increase the amount of stress. A few examples of negative reactions to stress to *avoid* are:

1. Avoidance
   - procrastination
   - skipping out
   - withdrawal
   - illness
   - sleep

2. Distractions
   - TV
   - socializing
   - video games
   - shopping

3. Violence
   - hurting others or yourself
   - throwing objects
   - yelling
   - hitting

4. Chemicals
   - smoking
   - sugar and caffeine
   - drugs and alcohol

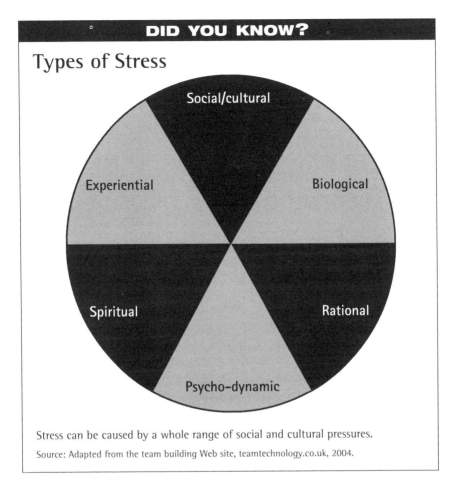

Types of Stress

Stress can be caused by a whole range of social and cultural pressures.

Source: Adapted from the team building Web site, teamtechnology.co.uk, 2004.

Negative coping strategies are typical reactions to stress and feelings of being overwhelmed. However, if a teen constantly use negative coping strategies, she or he can actually wind up causing more stress in the long run.

TYPES OF STRESS

Social cultural stress

Any major event in a person's life, good or bad, can be stressful. When a person's social circumstances change, such as loss of a parent, changing schools, or unwanted pregnancy, he or she might feel stressed. A person will experience stress when he or she is under pressure to conform to social patterns of behavior, especially where these behaviors are not the preferred behaviors of the individual, such as demands for cheating on exams, smoking, or drinking. When a person is experiencing conflicts in relationships or does not feel valued by others, he or she will feel stressed. Also, stress can be caused when a person feels he or she is not getting support from friends and family or that people do not want to listen to them. When a person does not have time to relax, he or she will often feel stress.

Biological stress

The causes of some stress lie in the biological makeup of your body or the interaction of your body with the food you eat or environment you live in. Some examples of the biological causes of stress include:

- lack of fitness
- poor diet such as a deficiency of vitamins; too much caffeine
- allergic reaction to chemicals in food
- genetic disorder resulting in chemical imbalances in the body.

Psychodynamic stress

The term *psychodynamic* refers to subconscious thoughts and feelings, which often arise from childhood experiences. The way in which you learned to cope in childhood was by using defense mechanisms that helped you manage the stresses you were experiencing. You still use those defenses today. Encountering situations that evoke stressful feelings that were experienced in childhood is one psychodynamic cause for stress. Spending time to maintain defenses in situations that threaten self-esteem and lack of self-awareness are other causes of stress.

Rational stress

The rational processes in our minds constantly interpret and evaluate the world around us. Events can be interpreted in many ways, and the way in which this is done can influence the level of stress that is felt. Perceiving the consequences of actions as being dangerous or threatening is a rational cause of stress. These perceptions may or may not be accurate—that is, the stress might be beneficial in preparing for a real danger, or harmful in creating unnecessary stress. Having an inaccurate perception of self and believing one is capable of achieving far too much, setting standards and expectations too high, and then failing is also stressful. When people misinterpret the actions of others so as to not accept the love and support that is given, they can experience stress. Not having the skill or knowledge to cope with certain situations, such as not having a rational approach to problem solving or conflict resolution, and therefore being unable to cope with problems as they arise will also cause a person to experience stress.

Experiential (that which is experienced) stress

The way in which each individual experiences each snapshot in time, even in very similar situations, is very different. One person may find a situation highly stressful, while another may find it stimulating or enjoyable; every reaction is unique. There may be many instant pressures that cause an individual to experience stress, such as too many demands from different people, as well as environmental stresses, such as noise, cramped conditions, or cluttered surroundings. When a person's needs are not met, he or she may become frustrated and feel stress. When there is a threat to survival, self-esteem, or identity, a person will also feel anxious. Changes in patterns of eating, sleeping, and relationships are also stressful.

Spiritual stress

The need for individual spiritual development has long been recognized by religion. It is only during the last 30 years that psychology has acknowledged the existence of a spiritual side to the individual. Some spiritual causes of stress include the violation of personal or religious moral code, contravention of accepted group practice, or violation of laws; the lack of spiritual development; an absence of truth such as self-deception and deception of others; the lack of a sense of personal agency or the failure to recognize and exercise choice; and the absence of a relationship with a higher being and lack of forgiveness.

See also: Alcohol, Drugs, and Suicide; Mental Illness and Suicide

FURTHER READING
Bickerstaff, Linda. *Stress.* New York: Rosen, 2007.
Culling, Katy Sara. *Dark Clouds Gather: The True Story About Surviving Mood Disorders, Eating Disorders, Attempted Suicide and Self-Harm.* London: Chipmunkapublishing, 2008.

Joiner, Thomas. *Why People Die by Suicide.* Cambridge, Mass.: Harvard University Press, 2005.

■ SUICIDE AND THE GAY, LESBIAN, BISEXUAL, AND TRANSGENDER COMMUNITIES

The nonheterosexual population and the prevalence of suicides. In a survey conducted by A. R. D'Augelli and colleagues, 42 percent of gay, lesbian, bisexual, and transgender (GLBT) youth studied had thoughts of suicide at some time in their lives. About 48 percent said that the suicidal thoughts were clearly related to their sexual orientation. In addition, 54 percent of the suicide attempts made by gay and lesbian youth occurred before parents knew of the youths' sexual orientation. A large number of gay and lesbian suicides occur between the ages of 16 and 21.

Part of the challenge in addressing suicide prevention in diverse populations is determining the circumstances under which diversity matters. Sexual orientation should not be relevant to the suicide prevention network's charge to decrease deaths by suicide. What is relevant is getting to the root of the matter.

According to the Centre for Suicide Prevention in Calgary, Alberta, Canada, more than half of the GLBT youth who attempted suicide did so before parents knew of their sexual orientation. Although there are limitations in the available data, it appears that GLBT youth are three times more likely to attempt suicide than their heterosexual counterparts. Also, the limitation occurs in completed suicides.

Those youth who are at greater risk for suicide are the ones who are least likely to reveal their sexual orientation to anyone. And suicide may be a way of making sure that no one ever knows. If their GLBT friends knew of the sexual orientation, they are not always inclined to "tell."

According to Kevin Berrill, director of the Anti-Violence Project of the national Gay and Lesbian Task Force, "The increased risk of suicide facing these youth is linked to growing up in a society that teaches them to hide and to hate themselves."

RISK FACTORS FOR GLBT YOUTH

There are many risk factors for young people in the GLBT communities. They include:

- hostile school environment (being rejected by heterosexual peers)
- physical and verbal victimization
- lack of support networks, including rejection from family
- sexual abuse
- homelessness
- drug abuse
- prostitution
- feelings of isolation
- family problems
- discrimination and homophobia
- conversion therapies (The American Psychiatric Association released a position statement that homosexuality is not a mental illness and that conversion therapies may be unethical in some situations.)

PROTECTIVE FACTORS

Factors that can help GLBT youth deal with their problems include: strong family support, social equality with unlimited legal protection (especially on the school grounds), GLBT support groups established in schools, and available mental health providers and counselors who are culturally competent.

OPPORTUNITIES FOR PREVENTION

In a study on sexual orientation and risk for suicide, J. Stephen MacDaniel, a professor at Emory University's School of Medicine, and his colleagues suggested that programs aimed at suicide prevention for those who have a different sexual orientation should also provide services for psychosocial adjustments, work at diminishing the effects of discrimination, and aggressively treat psychiatric problems and substance abuse **disorders** if these risk factors are present.

Suicide prevention should maintain a strong focus on youth since many studies found increased rates of suicidal behavior among adolescents and young adults. Studies have shown that prevention efforts should be focused. Some interventions should be directed at parents so they can help their children. Interventions should also focus on early adolescents for screening for suicidal thoughts. The use of peer-based interventions is also useful.

See also: Culture and Suicide; Stress and Suicide; Suicide Prevention

FURTHER READING

Dorais, Michel, and Simon L. Lajeunesse. *Dead Boys Can't Dance: Sexual Orientation, Masculinity, and Suicide.* Montreal: McGill-Queen's University Press, 2004.

Joiner, Thomas. *Why People Die by Suicide.* Cambridge, Mass.: Harvard University Press, 2005.

■ SUICIDE AND EATING DISORDERS

Suicide, the taking of one's own life, and suicidal thoughts are often prevalent among people who are suffering from compulsive obsessions with food or weight, the diseases known as eating disorders. The risk of suicide is increased when another **disorder** is present, such as alcohol abuse, **anxiety**, or mood disorders. According to Paola Miotto, an Italian psychiatrist who is an expert in this area, the more severe the eating disorder, the greater the likelihood that another psychiatric disorder is also present, coupled with hopelessness.

Patients with **anorexia nervosa**, self-imposed starvation, have a higher suicide rate than patients suffering from **bulimia nervosa**, which is characterized by overeating followed by purging. Anorexia is more common in teenagers, while bulimia is more often seen in women in their 20s. However, there is no set age limit for either of the two diseases. Here are differences between anorexia and bulimia based on the American Psychiatric Association's definition:

Anorexia Nervosa

- refusal to maintain weight that is over the lowest weight considered normal for age and height
- intense fear of gaining weight or becoming fat, even though underweight
- distorted body image
- in women, three consecutive missed menstrual periods without pregnancy

Bulimia Nervosa

- recurrent episodes of binge eating (minimum average of two binge-eating episodes a week for at least three months)
- a feeling of lack of control over eating during the binges
- regular use of one or more of the following to prevent weight gain: self-induced vomiting, use of laxatives or diuretics, strict dieting or fasting, or vigorous exercise
- persistent overconcern with body shape and weight

Some researchers suggest that the suicide risk is greater among anorexia patients because sufferers have developed a calming effect toward pain through experiences of starvation or self-injury that is linked to anorexia, in which they are more likely to use more severe or lethal methods in their suicide attempts. Others suggest that anorexia patients starve themselves because they are suffering from **depression** and not eating serves as self-medication. Depression in itself is a chronic risk factor for suicide.

TEENS SPEAK

I Was Anorexic

My senior year in high school, I was in the honor society, played field hockey and had lots of friends. You never would have thought anything was wrong, but I hated myself because I thought I was fat. I thought I'd never have a boyfriend or be truly happy unless I was thin.

It wasn't long before I became compulsive about counting calories. I carefully planned what I would eat for the week, skipping meals and exercising excessively whenever I thought I'd consumed too many calories. I took up to six laxatives a day. Even though I really missed eating the foods I used to love, it was all worth it when I'd get on the scale and see I had lost more weight. Friends would say how lucky I was to be thin, even though my period stopped, my hair fell out, and my face became wan and swollen. I used to count my ribs lying in bed at night.

Ironically, even though my anorexia started with a desire to attract boys, it soon made me lose interest in them. I couldn't stand the thought of someone getting close enough to me to look at or touch my body. I had one girl-friend who was really worried about me, but I refused to believe I had a problem. When my field hockey coach said that she thought I had a problem, I took it to heart but felt paralyzed and couldn't help myself.

One day I blacked out and ended up in the hospital. There was no avoiding that I was an anorexic. In the hospital, my mother was actually shocked to see how underweight I was. She used to be jealous of the "cute, skinny jeans" I could wear. The most important part of my recovery was emotional. My whole family went into therapy. My mother and I, in particular, worked hard to understand why my self-esteem was so low and how to improve it.

Unfortunately, I can't say the story ends there. My junior year in college I had a relapse. But that time, the signs were easier to recognize and I got help. It was like reliving an awful nightmare. But I slowly got better.

Treatment

Promising treatments for anorexia and bulimia are finally coming to light. The usual treatment since the 1970s has always been hospitalization for weight regain followed by psychotherapy. Presently, research reveals that a form of family therapy that enlists parents' help in getting their teenage daughters to eat again helps to strengthen the patient's feeling of independence. It is important for parents to work together with the patient and therapist as a team and help steer the developmental challenges of their teenager. Medication for depression of anorexics has also proved to be effective and allows the patient's weight to regain. Cognitive behavior therapy works with the unrealistically negative thoughts those with bulimia have about their appearance and guides them in changing eating behaviors.

See also: Gender and Suicide; Mental Illness and Suicide

FURTHER READING
Culling, Katy Sara. *Dark Clouds Gather: The True Story About Surviving Mood Disorders, Eating Disorders, Attempted Suicide and Self-Harm.* London: Chipmunkapublishing, 2008.

■ SUICIDE PACTS
See: Homicide and Suicide

■ SUICIDE PREVENTION
Stopping someone from committing or attempting to commit suicide, the taking of one's own life. Suicide is the most preventable death because most individuals do not want to die; they just want the pain to go away. Suicide prevention is any activity that reduces the burden of death by suicide, the problem of suicide attempts, and the affliction of suicidal behavior. It is an activity that concentrates on those factors that protect someone from suicidality.

Because suicide is a complex phenomenon, prevention is challenging. How does someone stop someone else from killing himself or herself? Prevention efforts should ultimately reduce risk factors and promote protective factors. In addition, prevention should address all levels that influence suicide: individual, relationship, community, and society. Effective prevention strategies are necessary to promote awareness. It takes a community-wide effort that must involve all sectors of the community. It is a mistake to delegate the effort to one sector, for instance the medical institutions within a community such as emergency rooms or psychologists and psychiatrists. No one sector of the community can prevent suicide—the community needs to be in it together.

Q & A

Question: What can we do if we think someone is suicidal?

Answer: It is important to show a potentially suicidal person that we care. We must directly ask the person if he or she is considering suicide. This shows that we are taking the person's feelings seriously and helps to establish if the risk for suicide is real. If you feel uncomfortable asking, it is important that you get someone else to ask. We need to listen to the person, without judgment and by showing empathy. If the person says he or she is considering suicide, we need to get help for that person by enlisting the help of professionals, whether a family doctor, a mental-health center worker, a 24-hour crisis line, or even a hospital emergency room nurse if the person is imminently at risk. Do not leave the person alone until he or she has received help, and do not agree to keep the person's plan a secret.

APPROACHES

The first approach would be to restrict the means. If guns are one of the major methods teens use to kill themselves, we need to limit the availability of firearms. The most common location for the incident of suicide by youth using a firearm is in the home. Families need to assess whether or not a gun should be in the home. Most families do not even realize their children know where the gun is located. This seemingly unmindfulness needs to be addressed. How important is it to have a gun in the home when there are teenagers in the house? And what are the chances of the gun being used to protect the family versus the gun being used by a family member to commit suicide? Restricting the access to a highly lethal means would allow for the suicide impulse to fade and perhaps diminish.

A second approach would be screening for **depression**. Children and young adults need to be screened for depression just as they are tested for other things such as eye exams, hearing tests, and dental checkups. Where untreated depression is one of the major causes of suicide, youth need to be examined for depression through screenings in which they would be asked to fill out a questionnaire—one or two pages—and depending on their responses, the examiner can determine if the youth is mildly suffering from depression or severely suffering from depression. These screenings should be mandatory.

A third approach is educational awareness. This is done through educational campaigns to educate groups of people and sectors of the community about suicide—the increasing rates, the causes, what to do in the event of a suicidal crisis, and basic general information on suicide, including the aftermath of suicide. Furthermore, it is essential to educate about the risk factors and protective factors so that families, schools, and community institutions can understand their roles in protecting teens against suicide and not contributing to the risk factors.

Q & A

Question: If someone really wants to kill himself, do you really think you can stop him?

Answer: Suicide is not about death. The person does not want to die; he or she is just trying to find a way to stop the pain. There is much ambivalence surrounding the decision to die by suicide, and by recognizing and discussing it, we can help the suicidal person start to recognize alternative options for managing their suffering. Often suicidal people are experiencing intolerable emotional pain, which they believe to be unrelenting. They feel hopeless and can see no other options. By helping them to see they have options, you are planting the seeds of hope that things can improve.

CRISIS HOTLINES

Hotlines provide counseling over the telephone if teens are in distress and feel they have nowhere to turn. They provide information as to where the nearest crisis center is located in the event they need immediate care. Hotlines provide a phone number people can call, generally at any time, and is answered by trained volunteers. Such hotlines have existed in most major cities of the United States at least since the mid-1970s. In the mid-1990s, a national 800 crisis line was created by Reese Butler, a man who lost his wife to suicide. He felt it was necessary to develop a hotline that people could use anywhere in the country and that was easy to remember—1-800-SUICIDE. This number still exists. However, after the creation of 1-800-SUICIDE, the government has now developed its own national crisis line, 1-800-273-TALK.

Crisis centers and hotlines offer 24-hour services to resolve crises of a suicidal nature. Teens feel that the anonymity and comfort of the telephone is better than direct face-to-face contact with a professional mental-health provider in the office or in an emergency room setting.

Talking on the phone is typically a little less formal and easygoing. Many counselors suggest the use of a hotline after hours if needed.

Q & A

Question: If a person's mind is made up, can she still be stopped from killing herself?

Answer: Absolutely. People who are contemplating suicide go back and forth, thinking about life and death. The pain often comes in waves. They don't want to die; they just want the pain to stop. Once they know they can be helped and there are treatments available for their illness—that it isn't their fault and that they are not alone—they find hope. We should never give up on someone just because we think she has made up her mind.

SCHOOL-BASED PROGRAMS

Many school-based programs are based on a gatekeeper training program in which those individuals who are constantly around the

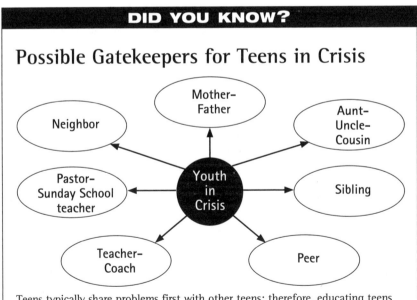

DID YOU KNOW?

Possible Gatekeepers for Teens in Crisis

Mother–Father

Aunt–Uncle–Cousin

Neighbor

Pastor–Sunday School teacher

Youth in Crisis

Sibling

Teacher–Coach

Peer

Teens typically share problems first with other teens; therefore, educating teens in using gatekeeper programs should have a positive effect so that teens as well as adults can help other teens in crisis.

Source: QPR Institute, 2008.

students on a daily basis (a gatekeeper) are trained to recognize when individuals are in suicidal crisis, how to restore them, and then get them the help they need. Gatekeeper training programs around the country include the LivingWorks Suicide Intervention based in Canada; Question, Persuade, and Refer (QPR) of Spokane, Washington; the Yellow Ribbon Training program out of Denver, Colorado; and many more. These national programs are offered all over the world. They demonstrate that motivated adults of any profession can be armed with enough information to save a life. These programs are often compared to CPR—where early recognition of signs are taught, then the application of knowledge, and finally the provision of help as soon as possible. The diagram below depicts the possible adults with whom a youth in crisis can interact many times throughout the day. These adults need to be trained as gatekeepers because when a youth is in crisis, he or she generally shows signs. These programs are skilled-based and action-oriented, designed to motivate adults to act fast when recognizing that a teen is in trouble. Adults learn critical facts regarding suicide and the associated warning signs.

SOS: SIGNS OF SUICIDE PROGRAM

The SOS (Signs of Suicide) Program for secondary schools, cosponsored by the National Association of Social Workers, is a program of mental-health screening and suicide prevention, which is implemented by school social workers during one or two school periods. The main teaching tool of the program is a video that teaches students how to identify symptoms of depression and suicidality in themselves or their friends and encourages students to seek help. The program's primary objectives are to educate teens that depression is a treatable illness and to teach them how to respond to a potential suicide in a friend or family member, using the SOS technique. SOS is an action-oriented approach instructing students how to ACT (Acknowledge, Care, and Tell) in the face of an emergency.

TEENSCREEN PROGRAM

The Columbia University TeenScreen Program in New York is committed to making the mental health of our youth a national priority and offering all parents the opportunity to have their teenagers receive a voluntary mental-health screening. The TeenScreen Program uses a questionnaire and interview process to see if a teen may be suffering from depression or other mental health problems. It is not a **diagnosis**. Treatment choices, if any, are left to parents.

Communities throughout the nation run their local screening programs with assistance from the National TeenScreen Program. Screenings take place in schools, doctors' offices, clinics, youth groups, shelters, and other youth-serving organizations and settings. While all local TeenScreen programs operate independently, they all adhere to the national program's implementation standards and requirements. Key among these is that screening is always a voluntary activity that requires both parent consent and teen agreement for participation.

TeenScreen focuses on screening for depression, anxiety, and alcohol and substance abuse because they are common, treatable conditions, and because most youths who suffer from them go undiagnosed and untreated. Research shows that a significant association exists between these **disorders** and suicide risk. Depression carries a particularly strong risk, with 60 percent of depressed teens thinking about suicide and 30 percent actually making suicide attempts. Although TeenScreen looks for the symptoms that are associated with different mental-health disorders, the program does not make any diagnoses and does not involve treatment.

SUICIDE SHOULD NOT BE A SECRET

In addition to learning the skills of taking action if a teen is in suicidal crisis, one of the most effective things that school-based programs instill is the importance of telling adults about a friend's suicidal thoughts—even if your suicidal friend wants you to keep it a secret. It is better to lose a friend and save a life. Tell someone, tell anyone, so that the suicidal teen can get the help that he or she needs.

Q & A

Question: What happens if a teen needs further evaluation after being screened through TeenScreen and does not have health insurance?

Answer: An important part of TeenScreen's development process is planning for needs like this. In order to be approved as a local TeenScreen program, relationships must be established with local health-care providers, including those that provide care at no cost or on a sliding scale basis. In addition, local programs must have the capacity to sign up uninsured youth for Medicaid and their state's

Child Health Insurance Program (CHIP). Many local TeenScreen programs also raise funds that enable them to provide scholarships to uninsured and underinsured teens.

According to the Canadian Mental Health Association, the beginning of the way out of life's troubles is to let someone else in. This is very hard to do because if a teen feels so desperate that suicide seems to be the only solution, he or she generally is frightened and ashamed. There is no reason to be ashamed of feeling suicidal and no reason to feel ashamed for seeking help. Teens are not alone; many people have felt suicidal when facing difficult times and have survived, usually returning to quite normal lives.

Teens need to take the risk of telling their feelings to someone they know and trust: a relative, friend, social service worker, or a religious leader. There are many ways to cope and get support. The sense of desperation and the wish to die will not go away at once, but it will pass. Regaining a will to live is more important than anything else at the moment. Hence, tell someone, tell anyone.

Some things to do if you have a friend who you think is suicidal:

- Listen without interrupting.
- Do not be judgmental.
- Do let him or her know that you care and you are on his or her side.
- Offer hope of any kind, such as saying, "We will get through this together."
- Offer to go with your friend to seek help from an adult.
- Let someone else who cares about this person know what is going on.
- Remember—if this person is talking to you—she or he has not fully decided to die yet. The person is still trying to decide.

WHAT TO DO FOLLOWING A SUICIDE ATTEMPT

A person may try to take his or her own life without warning or despite efforts to help. If you are involved in helping this person, make every effort to be calm and reassuring, and get medical help immediately. The time following an attempt is critical. The person should receive intensive care during this time. Maintain regular contact, and work with the person to organize support. It is vital that he or she does not feel cut off or shunned as a result of attempting suicide. Be aware that if someone is intent on dying, you may not be able to stop it from happening. You cannot and should not carry the responsibility for someone else's decision. Be mindful that all anyone can do is try.

Building strong coping skills

Dealing with death, depression, self-esteem, moving to a new school, **drug** dependency, peer pressure, the immigrant experience, body image, alcohol abuse, pregnancy, family problems, failure, or racism can take its toll on a teenager. School programs that demonstrate building good coping skills can decrease chances of students becoming suicidal. Helping kids learn how to cope with everyday issues by developing skills in communicating, problem solving, and relaxation is a step in the direction of good suicide prevention program.

See also: American Foundation for Suicide Prevention; Therapies and Psychodynamics

FURTHER READING

Alt, Jeff. *A Hike for Mike: An Uplifting Adventure Across the Sierra Nevada for Depression Awareness.* Cincinnati, Ohio: Dreams Shared Publications, 2005.

Collins, Christine, Ph.D., and Ron Salomon, M.D. *Suicide.* New York: Chelsea House, 2007.

Henden, John. *Preventing Suicide: The Solution Focused Approach.* New York: Wiley, 2008.

■ THERAPIES AND PSYCHODYNAMICS

Methods to prevent suicide by identifying individuals at risk and engaging them in clinical and professional treatment. There are three main types of therapies: (1) cognitive therapy, (2) psychodynamic therapy, and (3) behavioral therapy. All three types deal with thoughts, feelings, and behavior, with more emphasis on one while attempting to change the other. Cognitive therapies start with hopes of changing feelings and behavior. Psychodynamic therapy puts emphasis on how someone feels with the hopes of changing the thoughts and behavior. The behavioral therapist puts more emphasis on the behavior with hopes of changing the feelings and thoughts. Thoughts affect feelings, which affect behaviors. Thoughts, feelings, and behaviors interact with one another, and most therapies are known to use all three approaches. However, specific problems can have better results with a focus on one type of therapy.

WHY DO TEENS GO TO THERAPISTS?

It is always good for teens to talk about their feelings and thoughts, especially when they are going though bad times, either with family members, school, or friends. According to the Nemours Foundation's TeensHealth, when teens are going through these rough times and feeling sad, angry, or overwhelmed, they might feel supported if they talk to a therapist. A therapist can help sort out their feelings, finding solutions to their problems, or just help them feel better. Below are some reasons a teen may want to talk to a therapist:

- feels sad, depressed, worried, shy, or just stressed out
- dieting or overeating for too long or it becomes a problem (eating disorders)
- cuts, burns, or self-injures
- dealing with an attention problem (ADHD) or a learning problem
- coping with a chronic illness (such as diabetes or asthma) or a new **diagnosis** of a serious problem such as HIV, cancer, or a sexually transmitted disease (STD)
- dealing with family changes such as separation and divorce, or family problems such as alcoholism or addiction
- trying to cope with a traumatic event, death of a loved one, or worry over world events
- has a habit he or she would like to get rid of, such as nail biting, hair pulling, smoking, or spending too much money, or getting hooked on medications, drugs, or pills

- wants to sort out problems like managing anger or coping with peer pressure
- wants to build self-confidence or figure out ways to make more friends.

Therapy offers teens support to help them through difficult times. Deciding to seek help may be a teen's own decision, or it may come from a parent's or teacher's suggestion because they notice that the teen is dealing with a situation and they picked up some warnings that the teen may be in a crisis such as unexplained anger, sadness, losing or gaining weight, or not concentrating on studies coupled with a traumatic event. If a teen decided to seek help, or if someone decided for him or her, it is not a time to feel embarrassed or criticized or even unsure if it will work. It is a time for the teen to feel empowered because he or she is actually doing something about a situation that is affecting them.

PSYCHOTHERAPY

This is treatment usually given by a licensed psychologist or psychiatrist. It is different from counseling, which focuses on helping an individual solve normal problems. A counselor can range from someone with a degree in social work to someone who is certified to do counseling, but not necessarily a doctor. A psychologist is a nonmedical doctor with a Ph.D., an advanced degree. Psychologists who engage in psychotherapy generally do not prescribe medication but concentrate on a client's emotional state to help with changes in thoughts, feelings, and behavior. Psychiatrists have a medical degree (M.D.) and have completed advanced training in psychiatry. They can provide both psychotherapy and medication. Any change that happens while in therapy must come from within the person and his or her own efforts. Although a therapist can guide someone, no one can do the work for the patient.

Cognitive-behavioral therapy

This type of therapy emphasizes people's ability to make changes in their lives without having to understand why the change occurs. They focus on changing certain thought patterns, and by changing thought patterns behavior will also change.

Psychodynamic therapy

This type of therapy helps the client bring unconscious or hidden feelings to the surface. It is based on the assumption that feelings held in the unconscious mind are often too painful or uncomfortable to be realized. For that reason, people develop defense mechanisms to protect themselves from actually knowing about, dealing with, or confronting these feelings. Defense mechanisms are patterns of feelings that are unconscious. These mechanisms can be healthy or unhealthy but are a way to cope with the world. An example of a defense mechanism would be **denial**–refusing to face or perceive an unpleasant reality.

What happens in therapy?

A therapist will try to develop a relationship with you and build trust so as to help you discover what is going on and generally holds you in high regard because you are a person, no matter what your problem. Some of the goals in therapy include:

- improving self-esteem and gaining confidence
- figuring out how to make more friends
- feeling less depressed or less anxious
- improving grades at school
- learning to manage anger and frustration
- making healthier choices (for example, about relationships or eating) and ending self-defeating behaviors.

A session with a therapist generally lasts for one hour but can last longer for the first visit as a relationship begins to build. If someone is not able to build a good relationship and does not feel comfortable with the therapist, he or she should try another therapist. A person should pick a therapist the way you would pick a pair of shoes–there has to be a good fit in order to feel comfortable.

Q & A

Question: What is the link between mental health and suicide?

Answer: Up to 90 percent of people who die by suicide are suffering from some form of mental-health issue such as **depression,**

substance abuse, or other diagnosable disorders. Often this is not determined until after their death—by questioning family and friends as well as family physicians—because many of these people are never detected, assessed, or diagnosed. While the presence of a mental-health issue is strongly associated with suicide, it is important to note that most people with a mental-health issue do not die by suicide, and a mental-health issue does not singularly cause suicide.

You don't have to be *"crazy"* to seek help from a therapist
The word *crazy* can mean mentally deranged or demented. However, it is often used inappropriately and certainly has a **stigma** attached to it, just as *mental disorder* can also have a negative association. However, we need to make it perfectly clear that a stigma should not be attached to either term. Sometimes seeking help means you are overwhelmed with emotional stress. Getting help for emotional or stressful situations is as important to your overall health as getting help with a medical problem such as asthma or diabetes. Your mental state will sometimes need attending to just as a bad tooth will need filling. Emotional stress that becomes overwhelming and difficult to bear can cause psychological pain or a *psychache,* like a toothache. A therapist will get to the root of the psychological pain and discover whether the client is feeling disconnected or empty or worthless or hopeless or some other emotion that needs attention and treatment.

Crazy can mean irrational, impractical, or erratic, and choosing to seek help from a therapist is just the opposite. It means handling problems rationally and practically. You will not be ignoring your problems or hiding them, which only makes it worse. If you think that therapy could help you with a problem, ask an adult you trust, such as a parent, school counselor, or doctor to help you find a therapist.

Therapy is helpful to people of all ages and who have problems that range from mild to much more serious. Some people still hold on to old beliefs about therapy, such as thinking that teens "will grow out of" their problems. If the adults in your family don't seem open to talking about therapy, mention your concerns to a school counselor, coach, or doctor. You don't have to hide the fact that you're going to a therapist, but you also don't have to tell anyone if you'd prefer not to. Some people find that talking to a few close friends about their therapy helps them to work out their problems and feel like they're not alone. Other people choose not to tell anyone, especially if they feel that others won't understand. Either way, it's a personal decision.

Treatment with medication (psychopharmacology)

When is it appropriate to see a doctor who can prescribe medication? There is no antisuicide pill, but medication can be useful when there are chemical imbalances in the brain that are causing a major depressive illness. There is medication that will balance the chemicals and decrease the episodes of depression. These medications are known as antidepressants. Other types of mental disorders for which medication may be necessary or required are: **bipolar disorder,** for which mood stabilizers are prescribed; **anxiety disorder,** for which some mild tranquilizers may elevate the disorder; and **schizophrenia,** for which antipsychotics may be prescribed. All of the mentioned disorders are generally assessed by a psychiatrist, who is a medical doctor (M.D.). Psychologists (Ph.D.s) do not prescribe medication, nor does a general therapist. A discussion with a competent psychiatrist can help determine if medication is appropriate. Nevertheless, medication is seldom the only answer.

FURTHER READING

Alt, Jeff. *A Hike for Mike: An Uplifting Adventure Across the Sierra Nevada for Depression Awareness.* Cincinnati, Ohio: Dreams Shared Publications, 2005.

Henden, John. *Preventing Suicide: The Solution Focused Approach.* New York: Wiley, 2008.

■ WARNING SIGNS

Those signals that individuals give when they are in a suicidal crisis. A suicidal crisis occurs when a person is thinking and planning to take his or her own life or actually getting ready to attempt suicide. It is at this point that a person begins giving out all sorts of signs. Signals vary, and there is rarely just one signal, but several. Three main warning signs that need to be taken seriously include:

1) someone threatening to hurt or kill himself or herself, or talking of wanting to hurt or kill himself or herself; 2) someone looking for ways to kill him/herself by seeking access to firearms, available pills, or other means; and 3) someone talking or writing about death, dying, or suicide when these actions are out of the ordinary for the person.

OTHER BASIC SIGNS

The following signs tell us that a person may be in danger of thinking about suicide. Be aware if someone is exhibiting several of the signs listed below:

- abrupt changes in personality
- giving away possessions
- previous suicide attempt
- use of drugs and/or alcohol
- change in eating pattern, such as significant weight change
- change in sleeping pattern, such as insomnia or oversleeping
- unwillingness or inability to communicate
- **depression**
- extreme or extended boredom
- accident-prone (carelessness)
- unusual sadness, discouragement, and loneliness
- talk of wanting to die
- neglect of academic work and/or personal appearance
- family disruptions—divorce, trauma, losing loved one
- running away from home or truancy from school
- rebelliousness—reckless behavior
- withdrawal from people/activities they love
- confusion—inability to concentrate
- chronic pain, panic, or anxiety
- perfectionism
- restlessness

Q & A

Question: Is talking about suicide or threatening to do it just a ploy to get attention?

Answer: No. People who threaten to die by suicide mean what they say. People announce their intent to take their own life about 80 percent of the time, whether they are trying to make it sound like a joke or making a reference to being dead or giving other warning signs. They are letting us know what's on their mind, which is their way of asking for help. If they are looking for help, we need to give it to them.

Q & A

Question: Do people who attempt suicide do it to prove something, to show people how bad they feel, and to get sympathy?

Answer: They don't do it necessarily to prove something, but it is certainly a cry for help. This cry for help should never be ignored. This is a warning to people that something is terribly wrong. Many times people cannot express how horrible or desperate they are feeling and simply cannot put their pain into words. They can find no way to describe it. A suicide attempt must always be taken seriously. If they don't get the help for their underlying problem, people who have attempted suicide in the past may be at risk for trying it again and possibly completing it.

BE AWARE OF SOMEONE'S FEELINGS

Many teens at some point think about completing suicide. Most decide to live because they eventually come to realize that the feelings are only temporary and death is permanent. On other hand, people having a suicidal crisis sometimes perceive their dilemma as inescapable and feel a loss of control. These are some of the feelings and thoughts they may experience:

- can't stop the pain
- can't think clearly
- can't make decisions
- can't see any way out
- can't sleep, eat, or work

- can't get out of depression
- can't make the sadness go away
- can't see a future without pain
- can't see themselves as worthwhile
- can't get someone's attention
- can't seem to get control

If someone you know exhibits these symptoms, offer help, or contact someone close to the person!

IS THE PATH TO SUICIDE GETTING WARM?

Here is an easy way to remember these warning signs:

Is Path Warm

I   ideation (thinking about suicide)

S   substance abuse

P   purposelessness

A   anxiety

T   trapped

H   hopelessness

W   withdrawal

A   anger

R   recklessness

M   mood changes

The above-mentioned signs are considered warnings. Keep in mind too that some of them are coping strategies, as those exhibiting these strategies are trying to keep on living despite their feelings. Here are some ways to be helpful to someone who is threatening suicide:

- Be direct. Talk openly about suicide without passing judgment.
- Be willing to listen. Allow expressions of feelings. Accept the feelings.
- Do not debate whether suicide is right or wrong, or whether feelings are good or bad. Do not lecture on the value of life. Try to be as understanding as possible that these feelings exist.

- Get involved. Become available. Show interest and support.
- Do not dare someone to do it.
- Do not act shocked. This will put distance between you.
- Do not be sworn to secrecy. Seek support.
- Offer hope that alternatives are available, and do not make promises you cannot keep.
- Take action.
- Get help from persons or agencies specializing in crisis intervention and suicide prevention, such as a suicide prevention crisis center. Call 1-800-273-TALK (8255) for counseling as well as the nearest crisis center in your area. Also, be open to contacting a family physician, a private therapist or counselor, a school counselor or psychologist, or going to a community mental-health agency.

See also: Stress and Suicide; Suicide Prevention

FURTHER READING
Culling, Katy Sara. *Dark Clouds Gather: The True Story About Surviving Mood Disorders, Eating Disorders, Attempted Suicide and Self-Harm.* London: Chipmunkapublishing, 2008.
Henden, John. *Preventing Suicide: The Solution Focused Approach.* New York: Wiley, 2008.

HOTLINES AND HELP SITES

Active Minds
URL: www.activemindsoncampus.org
Phone: 1-202-332-9595
Programs: The young adult voice in mental-health advocacy on more than 100 college campuses nationwide
Mission: Peer-to-peer organization dedicated to raising awareness about mental health among college students

American Association of Suicidology
URL: http://www.suicidology.org
Phone: 1-202-237-2280
Programs: Promote research, professional and gatekeeper education, and suicide prevention; publishes two quarterly newsletters, one written for and by survivors of suicide; publishes the bi-monthly journal *Suicide and Life Threatening Behavior*

American Foundation for Suicide Prevention
URL: http://www.afsp.org
Phone: 1-212-363-3500
Programs: Dedicated to understanding and preventing suicide through research and education and to reaching out to people with mood disorders and those affected by suicide

Depression and Bipolar Support Alliance
URL: http://www.dbsalliance.org
Phone: 1-800-826-3632

Programs: Educational programs and events, e-newsletters, patient support groups, recovery education center, advocacy, reporting of research, and clinical trials

Mission: To provide hope, help, and support to improve lives of people living with depression or bipolar disorder

Families for Depression Awareness

URL: http://www.familyaware.org

Phone: 1-781-890-0220

Programs: Information and resources; Family Profiles, interviews with people coping with depression; community outreach; awareness workshops; advocacy

Mission: To help families recognize and cope with depressive disorders; to get people well and prevent suicide; help families recognize and manage various forms of depression and associated mood disorders; reduce stigma associated with depression; unite families and help them heal in coping with depression

The Jason Foundation

URL: http://www.jasonfoundation.com

Phone: 1-615-264-2323 or 1-888-881-2323

Programs: Offer staff development training for educators, school personnel, and youth workers. This training is available in several formats: staff presented, interactive CD-ROM, or DVD, and via the Internet. Since June 2007, JFI has averaged more than 2,700 individual training sessions each month, primarily to educators. In addition, JFI offers a Parent Resource Program (PRP) to educate parents about recognizing the signs of concern (warning signs), understanding elevated risk factors in youth, and how to respond effectively. "A Promise for Tomorrow" is JFI's school-based curriculum, which is designed for use in grades 7–12. It is a complete lesson plan for youth suicide awareness and prevention, including a teacher manual, discussion video, and PowerPoint CD. The program focus is the prevention of suicide by teaching recognition of signs of concern, providing peer support, and knowing appropriate responses to youth in crisis.

The Jed Foundation

URL: http://www.jedfoundation.org

Phone: 1-212-343-0016

Programs: HalfofUS.com; MTV's college network; Ulifeline, an online resource center with a screening tool; and campus-specific resources for more than 1,250 colleges

Mission: To prevent suicide and reduce emotional distress among college students

The Link's National Resource Center for Suicide Prevention
URL: http://www.thelink.org
Phone: 1-404-256-9797
Programs: Prevention and Aftercare, which are dedicated to reaching out to those affected by suicide and connecting them to the resources available
Mission: To provide a nonprofit community counseling center, which has been a national resource for suicide prevention and survivors of suicide for 30 years

National Institute of Mental Health (NIMH)
URL: http://www.nimh.nih.gov/
Phone: 1-301-443-4513
Programs: Support the science of brain and behavior as a foundation for understanding mental disorders; define genetic and environmental risk factors; develop tests and biomarkers for mental disorders; develop safe, effective, equitable treatments; support clinical trials; rapidly disseminate science information to mental health-care professionals and services
Mission: To reduce the burden of mental illness and behavioral disorders through research on the mind, brain, and behavior

National Organization for People of Color Against Suicide (NOPCAS)
URL: http://www.nopcas.org
Phone: 1-202-549-6039 or 866-899-5317
Programs: Prevention, intervention, and postvention support services to the families and communities affected adversely by the effects of violence, depression, and suicide in an effort to decrease life threatening behavior
Mission: To increase suicide awareness and education

National Suicide Prevention Lifeline
URL: www.suicidepreventionlifeline.org
Phone: 1-800-273-TALK

Mission: National crisis line that can be called from anywhere in the country and answered by trained professionals to help those in a suicidal crisis; available 24 hours

Samaritans USA (SAMS USA)
URL: http://www.samaritansusa.org
Phone: 1-212-677-3009
Programs: Coalition of the 10 community-based Samaritans suicide prevention centers in the United States
Mission: 1) To provide immediate and ongoing emotional support to those who are in crisis or have lost a loved one to suicide; 2) to teach lay and professional caregivers and service providers the most effective methods to prevent suicide; and 3) to educate caregivers, service providers, academics, those in government, industry, and the general public about the public health problem posed by suicide and the best means to prevent it

Suicide Awareness Voices of Education (SAVE)
URL: http://www.save.org
Phone: 1-952-946-7998
Mission: To prevent suicide through public awareness and education by developing public messaging campaigns and educational programs; reduce stigma and raise awareness of brain illnesses and their link to suicide; educate and train youth, adults, communities, and professionals; distribute prevention, grief support, and resources nationally and internationally; provide technical and professional assistance nationally

Suicide Prevention Action Network (SPANUSA)
URL: http://www.spanusa.org
Phone: 1-202-449-3600
Mission: To prevent suicide through public education and awareness, community engagement, and federal, state, and local grassroots advocacy; seeks to advance the implementation of the National Strategy for Suicide Prevention; envisions a world where suicide prevention is embraced as a public priority by all members of society

Yellow Ribbon Suicide Prevention Program
URL: http://www.yellowribbon.org
Phone: 1-303-429-3530

Programs: Task forces; Be-A-Link Gatekeeper; Ask 4 Help! Training for youth; Ask4Help cards; LifeSkills training; community development; and Yellow Ribbon curricula for schools, churches, workplaces, and the public in the United States, Canada, Australia, and other countries, and in tribal and native communities

Mission: To save lives from suicide through awareness, education, youth empowerment, prevention, and postvention work

GLOSSARY

acute a sharp, sudden, and severe pain or reaction

acute suicide threat a warning from an individual that he or she has the lethal means to commit suicide and voices the intent to do so

addiction a chronic, relapsing condition or disease characterized by compulsive alcohol, tobacco, or drug-seeking and abuse and by long-lasting chemical changes in the brain

adjustment disorder a mental condition characterized by depression or anxiety or combined depression and anxiety

adolescent suicide syndrome a disorder of youths characterized by impulsiveness, aggression toward self, or social loss

anniversary reaction the worsening of grieving on dates related to a loss

anorexia nervosa a psychiatric diagnosis that describes an eating disorder, which is characterized by self-imposed starvation, low body weight, body image distortion, and an obsessive fear of gaining weight

anticipatory grief grief felt in expectation of a loved one's death

anxiety disorder a mental disorder characterized by extreme and almost constant worry

assisted suicide   the completion of suicide with the aid of a physician or other health-care professional; illegal in the United States, except in Oregon and Washington

bipolar disorder   a brain disorder that causes extreme shifts in a person's energy, mood, and ability to function; also known as manic-depressive illness

bulimia nervosa   a psychiatric diagnosis that describes an eating disorder characterized by recurrent binge eating, followed by compensatory behaviors, referred to as "purging," or self-induced vomiting

chemical deficiency   an insufficient amount of a neurotransmitter, such as serotonin, within a person's brain

chronic grief   ongoing, acute grieving over time

chronic grief syndrome   the condition of an abnormal grief reaction after the loss of a deeply dependent relationship

chronically suicidal   a term used to describe someone who has a history of multiple suicide attempts

conduct disorder   a term used to describe a pattern of repetitive behavior where the rights of others or the current social norms are violated; symptoms often include verbal and physical aggression, cruel behavior toward people and animals, and other destructive behavior such as lying, stealing, truancy, and vandalism

delayed grief   bereavement that occurs years or decades after a loss

denial   refusal to accept the need for help or refusal to accept that a loss has occurred

depression   chemical imbalances in the brain that cause a mental disorder involving abnormal sadness and hopelessness; when severe, impairs normal functioning

diagnosis a clinical identification of the cause and nature of a condition, illness, or disease

disorder a clinically significant psychological or psychiatric condition

dopamine a brain chemical, classified as a neurotransmitter, found in regions of the brain that regulate movement, emotion, motivation, and pleasure

double suicide the completion of suicides by a couple or by two friends

drug a chemical compound or substance that can alter the structure and function of the body; psychoactive drugs affect the function of the brain, and some of these may be illegal to use and possess.

endorphins naturally occurring morphinelike substances found in the body

family history the presence of a disorder or risk factors in parents, siblings, or other family members

major depression when severe, a mental disorder, caused by a chemical imbalance in the brain, which impairs normal functioning; clinical depression

mass suicide the completion of suicide by an organized group; involving several people

medication a drug that is used to treat an illness or disease according to established medical guidelines

murder-suicide a situation in which the suicide victim commits homicide before completing the suicide

neurobiology the study of the brain and its physiology

neuron a brain cell that processes information

neurotransmitter   a neurochemical, such as serotonin, that attaches to a receptor in the brain to transfer signals between a neuron and another cell

panic attack   an episode of extreme anxiety; the recurring crisis phase of a panic disorder

post-traumatic stress disorder (PTSD)   an anxiety disorder characterized by a severe and recurring emotional reaction to a traumatic event, such as a violent assault or war

pseudocide   a pseudo-suicide; a faked suicide

schizophrenia   a mental disorder characterized by abnormalities in the perception or expression of reality; a loss of contact with reality

selective serotonin reuptake inhibitor (SSRI)   an antidepressant that acts on the chemical in the brain called serotonin and is used in the treatment of depression, anxiety disorders, and some personality disorders

serotonin   a neurotransmitter or chemical that inhibits self-destructive behavior

stigma   a socially unacceptable characteristic of a person, such as a disease or mental illness, which causes that person shame, to be looked down upon, or discriminated against

stressor   a factor or event that precipitates or drives a negative behavior or outcome

suicide contagion   a series of consecutive suicides

synapse   the point of connection between two nerve cells

terminal illness   a disease that inevitably ends with death

trigger   a factor or event that initiates and aggravates a specific behavior or a response

INDEX

Page numbers in *italic* indicate graphs or sidebars. Page numbers in **bold** denote main entries.